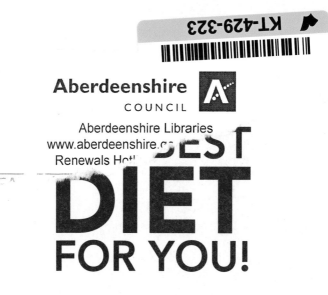

DIET FOR YOU!

THIS IS A CARLTON BOOK

Published in 2014 by Carlton Books Limited
20 Mortimer Street
London W1T 3JW

10 9 8 7 6 5 4 3 2 1

Text and Design © Carlton Books Limited 2014

A CIP catalogue record for this book is available
from the British Library.

ISBN 978 1 78097 448 4

Printed and bound in the UK by
CPI Group (UK) Ltd, Croydon, CR0 4YY

*This book reports information and opinions which may be of general
interest to the reader. It is advisory only and is not intended to serve as
a substitute for consultation with a physician. Be sure to get medical
advice from your doctor before embarking on any dietary programme.*

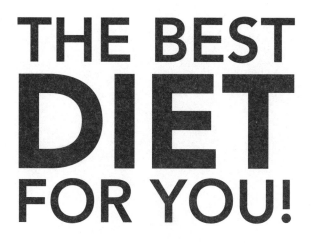

THE BEST DIET FOR YOU!

Caroline Jones

CARLTON
BOOKS

Contents

Foreword

Generally, for healthy weight loss, advice is to aim for a steady weight loss of about 1–2 lb (0.5–1 kg) per week. In practice this means reducing your calorie intake by about 500 kcal per day, which would mean consuming 1,500 kcal per day for an average woman. The theory of weight loss is, on the surface, very simple; anything that means you consistently consume fewer calories than you burn off will cause weight loss, and many of the weird and wonderful theories about how fad diets work simply boil down to the fact that you consume very few calories. However, healthy weight loss is not just about calories – it's also about the quality of the diet and making sure the food you eat is providing all the essential nutrients you need for good health. Balance and variety are key for a healthy diet and any weight loss plan that encourages the complete exclusion of several key foods or whole food groups (e.g. dairy foods, carbohydrate-containing foods) will put you at risk of missing out on vitamins, minerals and/or fibre, potentially storing up health problems.

Checking with your GP before starting a weight loss plan is a must for anyone with an underlying health condition, but is also not a bad idea even if you are not aware of any medical issues that might affect you. Conditions such as high blood pressure, high blood cholesterol or issues with blood glucose control can go undetected and can be important in choosing the best approach to weight loss. Diets that have a very high proportion of protein and those that encourage fasting or very low calorie intakes in particular may be risky if you are not in good health.

Anyone who has ever tried to lose weight can tell you that it is not easy – restricting our food intake in an environment where tasty, inexpensive food is readily available goes against thousands of years of our evolution. Sadly, research shows that of all those who lose weight, about 80 per cent will put the weight back within one year. Key barriers citied by slimmers include being hungry and restriction of foods.

Another big issue that we have to contend with when losing weight is our emotional wellbeing. In practice, no one chooses food and drink simply for its nutritional content and potential health benefits, our eating habits are influenced by a multitude of social and psychological factors. Food, especially the energy dense foods that we typically need to cut down when dieting, provides an emotional reward that we are naturally drawn to and constantly having to avoid such foods can make us feel deprived. Add to this all the negative perceptions around overweight and obesity in our society and it's clear that for many, losing weight will be emotionally as well as physically challenging.

If this all sounds overly negative, then the good news is that research shows that people can lose weight and keep it off in the long term. One factor that successful slimmers have in common is that they exercise "flexible restraint", that is, they watch what they eat but don't completely exclude the foods they like and they are not thrown by small slips-ups in their diet plan. They tend to be physically active and, perhaps just as importantly, don't spend a lot of time in sedentary activities such as watching TV. The tend to eat a relatively low fat diet, which will mean that they can eat satisfying portions of food – key to keeping you feeling full and avoiding feeling deprived. They eat breakfast and maintain a structured eating plan, both during the week and at the weekends and regularly monitor their weight. While there is no "one size fits all" or magic bullet when it comes to weight loss, keeping these principles in mind may help when choosing the right plan for you. Ultimately, most people will only be able to keep up any out-of-the-ordinary eating pattern for a relatively short time in order to reach a weight loss goal. The real challenge, once you've lost the weight is to maintain that weight loss. However, by making sustainable changes to your diet and lifestyle, you can keep the weight off for life.

Bridget Benelam
Senior Nutrition Scientist, British Nutrition Foundation

Introduction

Research reveals that six in every 10 women admit to desperately wanting to lose weight – that's more than half of the female population counting calories or simply saying no to treats on daily basis.

With weight such a universal worry, is it any wonder many of us are prepared to try any diet we hear works in an attempt to achieve our goal? But with so much conflicting advice out there, and so many weight-loss options, how on earth do you know which diet is the right one for you? The choice can be overwhelming.

Take a quick glance at any magazine stand or bookshop shelf and you'll be bombarded with the latest and greatest weight-loss cures, from diets that trim fat or cut out carbs to those that push new superfoods or fasting days. Indeed, every year yet another celebrity diet craze sweeps the nation. And some of us seem in vain to try them all! In fact, researchers estimate that the average woman wastes a worrying 30 years of her life struggling to shed pounds on a diet.

The problem is, a "one-size-fits-all" approach doesn't work with dieting. So being the first to jump on the latest fad or following the advice of others – even if they are famous – is no guarantee of weight-loss success. You probably know from bitter experience that just because your best friend shed 20 lb (9 kg) with WeightWatchers, for example, it doesn't mean you'll do the same. And while your favourite movie star might swear by the Blood Type diet, the chances are you'll find the scales don't go in your favour, despite slavishly following it.

The truth that the hugely profitable diet industry prefers to keep secret is that a whole lot of time, money and stress could be saved if only there was a method to help match a diet to everything that is unique about you. Which is where this handy book comes in. The volume you're holding in your hands is not another diet book – the world has too many of them already! Instead it's an easy-to-digest guide to the best, biggest (and in some cases baddest) diet plans, so you don't have to become an expert on them all yourself. In the coming pages you will find a comprehensive look at the top 30 modern diets,from Dukan to Detox, outlining their general philosophy, their history and their eating and exercise plans. We then take a

Dieting through the Decades

1000 BC	1820	1860s
The Moderation Diet	**The Vinegar and Water Diet**	**The Banting Diet**
The ancient Greeks followed a policy of moderation, practising a good balance of eating, exercising and sleep. They were very knowledgeable about health and diet and observed that over-weight men suffered from unhealthy hearts.	In order to cleanse and purge his body, the poet Lord Byron would drink vinegar daily and eat potatoes soaked in the stuff. Side effects included vomiting and diarrhoea. Unsurprisingly this extreme regime left him with numerous health problems.	Probably the first low-carb diet. William Banting's pamphlet *A Letter on Corpulence, Addressed to the Public in 1863* outlined a strict low-carbohydrate, low-calorie diet that the formerly obese English undertaker had used to shed an impressive 46 lb (21 kg) in 12 months after becoming too fat to tie his own shoe laces.

more critical look at the pros and cons of each plan, assessing their suitability for your body type, personality and lifestyle. We will also highlight where the science is shaky and any hidden health concerns. All of which means you won't have to spend such a large chunk of your life trying all of them out!

The guidance in this book will not only ensure you make the right diet choice to achieve successful weight loss, it will hopefully help you find a healthy eating plan you can comfortably sustain for a lifetime.

It's All Greek: A Potted History of Dieting

If you thought dieting was a particularly modern obsession, think again. The roots of the term dieting, literally "the practice

Dieting through the Decades continued

1900

The Chew Chew Diet

Horace Fletcher, an American entrepreneur, had become so fat he was refused life insurance. Determined to lose weight he created Fletcherism, or the "Chew Chew" diet as it was called, which promoted chewing a mouthful of food until all "goodness" was extracted, then spitting out the fibrous material that was left. He lost over 40 lb (18 kg) on the plan and gained the nickname the Great Masticator, with his radical diet becoming hugely popular.

1920s

The Calorie Counting Diet

The 1920s fashion for thin, boyish figures for women helped lead to the popularity of counting the number of calories in food to lose weight. Doctor Lulu Hunt Peters published *Diet & Health: With Key to the Calories* in 1918. It sold millions of copies, becoming the first diet bestseller. She urged women to view food as calories, and not to consume more than 1,200 a day.

of eating food in a regulated fashion to decrease body weight", go back as far as the ancient Greeks. But in those days diatia, the Greek word from which "diet" is derived, described an entire holistic body and mind approach to life, which encouraged moderation in everything – not just food and drink – to ensure happiness and good health.

Dieting with the sole aim of shedding excess pounds didn't become a widespread practice until the 1800s, mainly because it was relatively unusual to be overweight. Unless you were a successful merchant, a wealthy cleric or a member of the aristocracy, you simply didn't have access to enough food to grow particularly corpulent. The super-obese epidemic we're experiencing today is largely due to the abundance of cheap, high-calorie food. But go back

1930s

The Hay Diet

This diet, established by American Doctor William Hay, was based on the idea that food was either protein, starch or neutral – protein and starch, he believed, should not be eaten in the same meal. Famous followers included car manufacturer Henry Ford.

1940s

The Master Cleanse Diet

Nutrition guru Stanley Burroughs created the Master Cleanse, a fast during which the dieter subsists solely on a mixture of cayenne pepper, fresh-squeezed lemon juice, maple syrup and water. It's still popular today, despite the fact that most nutritionists agree it's unsafe.

1950s

Cabbage Soup Diet

The creator is unknown, but the popularity of this gruelling diet has endured to the present day. It's usually a seven-day diet plan, consisting of mainly cabbage soup, supplemented with fruit and vegetables and a small amount of meat.

in time to 200 years ago, when food was scarcer and life physically tougher and more active, and it comes as no surprise that people were a good deal slimmer. Famously fat historical figures such as King Henry VIII – who by the age of 50 weighed 30 stone (420 lb/190.5 kg) and had a waist that measured a whopping 52 in (32 cm) – were both the exception and exceptionally privileged.

As one of the early "pretty boy" pin-ups, it is perhaps fitting that Romantic poet Lord Byron is credited with starting one of the first ever diet crazes in the early 1800s. Byron had an unfortunate propensity for gaining weight, fluctuating from a portly 14 stone (196 lb/89 kg) at his heaviest down to a rake-thin 9 stone (126 lb/57 kg). So in a bid to maintain the fashionable "pale and gaunt" look of the Romantic period,

Dieting through the Decades continued

1963	1972	1980
WeightWatchers	**The Atkins Diet**	**The Pritikin Diet**
The famous point system that allows you to lose pounds along with fellow WeightWatchers members was founded in the 1960s by Jean Nidetch, a self-described "overweight housewife obsessed with cookies".	Robert Atkins devised this high-protein diet based on his own weight-loss experiments, and in 1972 published *Dr Atkins' Diet Revolution*, which would go on to sell tens of millions of copies. Thirty years later in 2002, his follow-up book, *New Diet Revolution*, made the Atkins Diet more popular than ever.	Founded by Nathan Pritikin in the 1970s, but becoming popular in the early 1980s, this diet was one of the first "heart-friendly" low-fat, low-salt, high-fibre plans. Pritikin was an American engineer who became interested in nutrition after he was diagnosed with advanced heart disease aged 41. Before his death in 1985 he was regarded as a diet guru.

the poet extolled the virtues of a "potato and vinegar diet" for keeping the weight off.

Given his standing as a hugely famous and influential figure, Bryon was widely criticized for setting a terrible example to the young and impressionable. As one doctor at the time wrote: "Our young ladies live all their growing girlhood in semi-starvation [for fear of] incurring the horror of disciples of Lord Byron."

However it was not until several decades later that the Victorians, indulging their love of the extreme and quirky, helped kickstart the fad diet with a vengeance. Indeed, one of the earliest low-carb diet crazes to reach a major audience was published by undertaker William Banting in 1863. So important was its influence that "I'm banting" became a

1997	2000s	2013
The Blood Type Diet	**The Dukan Diet**	**The 5:2 Diet**
In *Eat Right for Your Type*, Peter D'Adamo, a naturopath, claimed that people should eat foods compatible with their blood type. Despite a lack of scientific backing, the diet soon became a celebrity favourite.	A French general practitioner, Pierre Dukan, developed his diet in the 1970s as a way of treating obese patients. But it was only in 2000, when he published his book in France that the low-carb, high protein Dukan Diet became more popular.	The 5:2 Diet or "fasting diet", which involves eating normally for five days and severely restricting calories on two non-consecutive days, is the most recent diet trend. As with many modern plans there are even claims it can reduce the risk of cancer and heart disease.

popular expression to mean, "I'm on a diet" – the use of which continued well into the 1920s.

The deprivations of successive world wars and economic depression barely interrupted the rise of fashionable slimming and by the post-war boom years there was simply no stopping the growing diet industry. New weight-loss plans arrived ever faster, from WeightWatchers and Atkins right up to today's Dukan Diet and 5:2 fasting plan. As a species, we've now tried just about every possible way to lose weight – and made the plans' creators very rich in the process. The business of dieting is now an unstoppable global industry that, despite the latest worldwide recession, is showing no signs of decline.

How safe – or indeed effective – many of these diets are has attracted much criticism from the scientific and medical communities over the years. Today there are lots of conflicting expert opinions to wade through and as many diet doubters as fans. But with obesity now officially a modern epidemic, the influx of exotic new ways to shift excess weight continues to grow at the same rate as our ever-expanding waistlines.

Ironically after 2000 years of trying extreme diets, from the eccentric to the downright dangerous, the latest research now suggests the ancient Greeks may have had the best solution all along. The Greek philosopher Socrates once said that "everything in moderation, nothing in excess" was the key to health and happiness and today most dieticians will agree that a moderate diet and exercise plan, a holistic diatia in other words, is the best way to stay at the right weight your whole life through. In addition, the traditional Greek/Mediterranean diet is now seen as probably the world's healthiest food plan. Indeed, the ancient Greeks even practiced their own form of the most recent diet trend: periodic fasting to help rest the body and keep weight down. Perhaps we should have listened to them all along!

But one way in which modern science has advanced our understanding of weight control is in new techniques to help determine which diets suit which person best. Development of both personality and gene testing means we're close to being able to create a totally bespoke diet plan that promises to fit with your physiology, personality and lifestyle. And if there's one thing nutrition experts tend to agree on, it's that for a diet to be successful it must be a good match for the individual.

In the future, for the right price, each of us will be able to obtain a DNA and character-matched diet plan tailored to our every personality quirk and specific biological need. But in the meantime, narrowing down your choice from the currently available diets with the help of this book is a good place to start. After all, regardless of the plan you eventually choose, if you have made a better-informed diet decision, you will see better, longer-lasting weight loss results – which is what we really want in the end.

The 5:2 Diet

2013's diet craze: fast for two days a week and feast on whatever you like for the rest of the time.

The weight-loss promise
Lose around 1 lb (450 g) a week as a woman, 1–2 lb (450–900 g) as a man. Plus, you will enjoy a wide range of health benefits, including improvements in blood pressure, cholesterol levels and insulin sensitivity.

Interestingly the popular "5:2" Diet approach of fasting for two days every week was originally developed by cancer doctors to help their patients endure chemotherapy. When the body doesn't have food, normal cells go into survival mode by slowing down and "hibernating". This means the fasting element of the diet can help to protect healthy cells against the effects of chemotherapy, which means fewer side effects.

In August 2012, the 5:2 Diet hit the mainstream and became something of an overnight sensation after featuring in a BBC documentary called "Eat, Fast and Live Longer" by health journalist Dr Michael Mosley. After just five weeks on the diet plan, Mosley lost nearly a stone (14 lb/6 kg), reduced his body fat by about 25 per cent and improved his blood sugar and cholesterol levels. Mosley's interest in intermittent fasting is highly personal. His father died aged 73 of complications related to type 2 diabetes, a disease linked with being overweight. So when Michael was diagnosed as pre-diabetic he tried out various intermittent fasting diets, having heard that they potentially had beneficial effects on insulin levels. He found the 5:2 approach to be the most effective.

The plan

The premise behind the diet is to "fast", or severely restrict calories, for two non-consecutive days a week and eat normally on the other five days. On fasting days, you must reduce your calorie intake to one quarter of your usual intake. For men this means 600 kcals, and for women 500. Success also depends on not over-eating during the five days of normal eating. You should eat sensibly – within guidelines of 2,000 calories a day for women and 2,500 for men – but you do not have to deny yourself anything, so if you want cake for dessert, you can have it.

Exercise

Some variations of the diet advise keeping to the UK government recommendations for exercise – 30 minutes, three times a week – on non-fasting days. Michael Mosley himself, however, seems to be more of an advocate of High Intensity Training (HIT), which involves short bursts of very intense exercise.

How it works

The rationale behind the 5:2 Diet centres on the effects that fasting has on levels of a hormone called IGF-1 (insulin-like growth factor 1). Although the hormone is essential in early life when rapid new cell growth is important, high levels in adulthood increase the risk of cell divisions such as those found in cancer. Restricting the calories you consume, so the theory goes, lowers blood levels of IGF-1, protecting you against some major diseases while also allowing you to burn fat at a higher rate and regulate blood sugar levels.

Taking your calorie intake down to such a low level also makes the body's organs work harder and more efficiently, and by spacing out the fasting days you avoid slipping into starvation mode – something that is believed to cause the body to store more fat. Some research suggests that your body goes into repair mode when it isn't getting any food, because it isn't having to use up all its energies on the digestion process. Through trial and error, Mosley found fasting for two days a week was both achievable and had the best results.

Mosley's book, *The Fast Diet*, became the UK's best-selling non-fiction book in February 2013, and the diet's popularity quickly spread from the UK to Europe and the USA. Advocates of the diet even claim it may increase lifespan and decrease the risk of conditions such as cancer and Alzheimer's disease. A host of celebrities are since said to have had success with it.

DAILY MENU EXAMPLE

Fasting Days
The 500 or 600 kcal limit requires small portions, as shown in the example below, and only water, black coffee and green tea to drink.

Breakfast	1 poached egg on half a slice of wholemeal toast spread with one grilled (broiled) tomato
Lunch	Tzatziki with cucumber and red pepper sticks
Dinner	Sweet potato soup (no bread)

PROS	CONS
• As you are restricting your calorie intake for only two days a week, you can still enjoy having meals out and drinks with friends on the other days, including at the weekends.	• Intermittent fasting is NOT suitable for pregnant or breastfeeding women.
• No food is banned on non-fast days, so it's easier to find the willpower to stick to the calorie restrictions on fasting days.	• Some people have reported difficulties sleeping, irritability and headaches.
• You don't have to splash out on expensive diet products. Your weekly food bill will actually be cheaper, as you'll be eating less two days a week!	• You'll need to think about how fasting will impact on your life. You will be very hungry and have less energy on the days that you fast, and you may find some of your regular activities are harder to accomplish.
	• On fasting days you are unlikely to meet the recommended daily amounts for many vital nutrients.

Who is it best for?

Lifestyle: You have a busy social life and you don't want your diet to stop you enjoying meals out and weekends away.

Personality: The diet suits those who struggle with willpower and have struggled in the past with sticking to rigid eating plans for the long term. You may also be curious about the latest craze and a keen follower of fashions.

Body shape: Pear shapes that carry most of their excess weight below the hips. Weight loss achieved by following a very low-fat, low-calorie diet often sees a reduction in fat from the breasts, shoulders and arms, but not from the thighs and buttocks, but this diet promises to reach those problem areas.

Any health concerns?

It's early days, so there isn't enough firm scientific evidence to prove claims that the 5:2 Diet helps people lose weight or boosts health in the long term, especially as, currently, most of the research has been done on rats rather than people. On the fasting days, because you're eating only a quarter of the calories you need, you may suffer from low blood sugar, and unless you increase your water intake, you could experience constipation. As you will be low on vitamin and mineral intakes on fast days, you need to focus on eating nutrient-rich foods on normal days to make up the shortfall. Also, intermittent fasting is not suitable for pregnant or breastfeeding women and for people with pre-existing health conditions, such as diabetes, or with a history of eating disorders. Before trying out this diet, and in fact any diet, especially one that involves periods of very low-calorie intake, it's important to talk it over with your doctor first.

Want to know more?

Read: *The Fast Diet: The Simple Secret of Intermittent Fasting* by Dr Michael Mosley and Mimi Spencer (Short Books, 2013).

The 5-Factor Diet

A celebrity favourite that breaks diet and exercise down into bite-sized chunks.

The weight-loss promise

"My revolutionary five-week programme will help you lose weight and get fit without feeling hungry or deprived – and is one of the easiest programmes to follow."

Harley Pasternak

This low-GI diet is the creation of Harley Pasternak, a Hollywood-celebrity fitness trainer who can count Halle Berry, Alicia Keys and Jennifer Hudson among his clients. Pasternak apparently wanted to create a diet and exercise programme that would comfortably fit into the on-set breaks of the celebrities he worked with. He says his clients' hectic schedules and lack of open space forced him to create The 5-Factor Diet, turning limited time, space and food into tools for success. "It requires the least amount of time for the most results – and that's exactly what my clients are looking for," he says.

Despite the fast results, it's not a crash diet. Pasternak doesn't believe in women becoming super-skinny – either for their looks or for their health. "If you're emaciated skinny, you don't feel great," he explains. "Women should look like women. They need natural curves, and if they're too lean, their hormonal cycle gets thrown off and they stop looking and feeling like women."

The plan

The number 5 is the key to this diet, which consists of five meals per day and five key ingredients at each meal. The five ingredients should be a healthy combination of protein, complex carbohydrates, fibre, fat and fluids. You should eat one mini meal every three to four hours. Each should include:

1. **A low-fat protein:** chicken breast, fish, shellfish, egg whites or cottage cheese.
2. **Healthy carbohydrates:** beans, lentils, brown rice, wild rice, fruit.
3. **Fibre:** from healthy carbs such as beans, oats, lentils, barley, brown rice, wholegrain bread, vegetables (except potatoes) and fruit.
4. **Healthy fats:** cooking oils such as olive and rapeseed (no full-fat dairy).
5. **A sugar-free drink**

In order to help you keep on the wagon and focused, the diet also allows for one "cheat" day each week on which you are allowed to eat whatever you like.

Exercise

The diet also includes an exercise regime, which consists of five specific exercises to be done for five minutes each, five days of the week – this works out at 25 minutes per session. Pasternak believes that working out more often for shorter periods of time is more effective than spending hours at the gym. Activities he recommends include running, cycling, dancing, brisk walking or swimming. For Pasternak, it is the variety that's key.

DAILY MENU EXAMPLE	
Breakfast	French toast: 2 slices of bread dipped in egg whites, skimmed milk and a little sugar, then grilled (broiled) and topped with low-fat ricotta cheese and a few berries
Snack	Turkey slices with celery dipped in homemade houmous
Lunch	Baked sweet potato with tuna
Snack	Edamame beans
Dinner	Seafood and vegetable stir-fry with rice noodles

How it works

The five-week programme combines balanced, healthy eating with particular emphasis on low-GI foods. Pasternak's premise is that low-GI foods help regulate insulin production, which helps control appetite and therefore promote weight loss. Pasternak claims his plan will keep blood sugar from spiking and dipping erratically and therefore stave off hunger. There is currently no scientific evidence to prove that eating five meals a day or eating GI food helps in weight loss. But the diet also effectively promotes the tried-and-tested weight-loss method of cutting total daily calories, eating healthier foods in moderation and following a regular exercise programme.

PROS	CONS
• It's a fast-working plan that promises results.	• Some people may find it tough to fit eating every 3–4 hours into their schedule.
• It promotes exercise, which is a healthy way to lose weight.	• The food plan incorporates cuisines from all around the world, which means some of the ingredients may be both hard to source and expensive.
• It encourages you to cook your own meals from scratch, rather than rely on convenience meals.	
• You're allowed a cheat day each week, which can help you stay motivated and stick to the diet for the rest of the week.	• The menu is the same for everyone regardless of your weight, gender or activity level.
	• The diet does not address what happens when you eat out.

Who is it best for?

Lifestyle: Those who have time to plan what they eat the night before, but have a busy daily schedule to get through.

Personality: You like to have clear, simple rules to stick to and have a strong sense of order and routine.

Body shape: Apples and pears who need the cardio exercise recommended on the plan to really help shift those particularly stubborn fat pockets around the tummy or hips.

Any health concerns?

There is nothing particularly dangerous about this diet. It's a solid and sensible approach to weight loss, which should help most people to lose weight. It doesn't ban any food groups or suggest eating dangerously low levels of calories. If followed correctly, the average person can expect some weight loss, at least in the short term, due to smaller meal sizes and the additional exercise. But, in the long term, the weight will only stay off if the dieter changes his or her eating habits for the better permanently.

Want to know more?

Read: *The 5-Factor Diet: Get the Body You Want in Just Five Weeks!* by Harley Pasternak with Myatt Murphy (Meredith Books, 2007).

The 17-Day Diet

A high-protein diet that promises super-fast results.

The weight-loss promise:
"A simple plan that targets both belly fat and visceral [intra-abdominal] fat and produces fast results that last, this diet promises a weight loss of up to 12 lb (5.4 kg) in just three weeks – all by activating your so-called 'skinny gene'."

Dr Mike Moreno

This fast-results diet was created by family GP Dr Mike Moreno, based in San Diego in the United States, as a way of helping his overweight patients shape up. The 17-Day Diet then became popular around the rest of the world when Moreno's book outlining the weight-loss plan was published in 2011. But it was on the internet that its fame really took off. In fact it's been credited as the first diet to go truly "viral", after followers who'd lost weight on the plan started posting video testimonies on YouTube and social-networking sites. This interest meant the diet appeared in the top 20 most searched-for words on Google for many weeks to follow.

The plan

Moreno's plan contains high amounts of low-fat protein sources, such as chicken, fish and lean meats. It's also packed with fruit and veg, but certain varieties of fruit, such as pineapple, watermelon and banana, are deemed too high in sugar and best avoided. It also recommends swapping "bad carbs", such as white bread, white rice and pasta, for "good" carbs, such as veg and whole grains. Throughout the plan, dieters are encouraged to exercise portion control, eat breakfast, pack in lots of salads, choose healthy substitutes, listen to when their bodies tell them they are hungry, eat slowly and drink plenty of water. The diet is broken into four cycles to be worked through one by one, each lasting the magic 17 days:

Cycle 1: Accelerate: Dieters clean up their diets, getting rid of fast foods, sugar and white carbs to promote rapid weight loss. This phase, Moreno says, is designed to "improve digestive health, help clear sugar from blood to boost fat-burning and discourage fat storage".

Cycle 2: Activate: This stage "resets your metabolism by increasing and decreasing calorie intake to stimulate fat burning". As in cycle 1, carbs are restricted after 2 p.m. The idea is to keep alternating between cycles 1 and 2 until you reach your goal weight.

Cycle 3: Achieve: Once you've lost the required weight, you can follow a more relaxed meal plan that reintroduces foods in sensible portions, along with one alcoholic drink per day. Expect weight loss to slow down unless you forgo alcohol and/or increase aerobic exercise.

Cycle 4: Arrive: This phase is all about maintenance and you're now allowed to enjoy up to three favourite meals during weekends.

Exercise

You're told to walk for 17 minutes a day during the first two cycles – no more because of the limited calorie intake. In the later cycles, you have to ramp up the exercise to 150–300 minutes per week for continued weight loss.

How it works

Dr Moreno says his diet's four phases are meant to "confuse" the body's metabolism. He chooses 17-day periods of dieting because he believes they keep the body's metabolism working as hard as possible, so that you burn off the maximum fat. "Day 17 is just before the time when your body starts to recognize the diet as an ongoing habit and your metabolism starts to slow as a result," he claims. By never allowing the body to adjust to new eating and exercise regimes, dieters avoid stubborn weight-loss plateaus, he adds. "With each 17-day cycle, you're changing your calorie count and the foods you eat. By varying these things, you prevent your body from adapting."

Dr Moreno defends his speedy diet plan from critics of crash diets. "Rapid weight loss can be safe if done correctly, and new research suggests that the faster you take weight off, the faster you keep it off – my diet is designed to produce quick results, not because it starves you, but because it's a carefully designed balance of food and exercise that adjusts your body so you burn fat, day in and day out."

Who is it best for?

Lifestyle: You're someone who can fit in all the extra shopping and preparation time, and probably don't have kids – unless you want to be preparing a different meal for the rest of the family every night. It's also better for a low to moderate exerciser, as in the early stages you don't consume enough calories for serious fitness fans.

Personality: A "doer" who likes quick fixes and fast results.

Sample day from Cycle 1

Unlimited lean protein

Unlimited non-starchy vegetables

2 low-sugar fruits

2 probiotics (low-fat yogurt)

1–2 servings of friendly fats (heart-healthy monounsaturated fats such as olive oil and nut or seed oils)

Green tea

2 litres of water

Body shape: People with big bellies, in particular, as Dr Moreno says this is where people on his diet will shift the weight from first.

Any health concerns?

This diet cuts out certain food groups and, in many cases, it's hard to try and make up for those lost calories by eating more of other foods groups – which is the main reason why you lose weight on any restrictive diet. With no cereal-based foods, your diet is likely to be low in fibre which could lead to constipation. Also, the downside of losing weight quickly,

PROS	CONS
• It gives quick results.	• It can be hard to follow without carrying the book around so you know which foods from the various food groups you can actually eat in your current cycle.
• Alternating cycles stop you getting bored.	
• If you want to kick-start a healthier diet, it can help you get on track.	• The total daily calorie during cycle 1 is low for some people, particularly if you're reasonably active.
• You'll probably be eating more fruit and veg with each meal than normal so your levels of disease-fighting antioxidants such as vitamins C and E will be higher.	• Although you're eating lots of fruit and veg, they have to be ones Dr Moreno deems to be "low-sugar", which will limit your choice a fair amount.

as on this plan, is that unless you intend to follow the diet permanently you will probably regain the weight you lost just as quickly. It's also worth bearing in mind that although following this diet for a short time could help kick-start your weight loss, staying on it for too long could mean you miss out on some of the key nutrients needed to stay fit and healthy.

Want to know more?

Read: *The 17-Day Diet* by Mike Moreno (Simon & Schuster Ltd, 2011).

The Atkins Diet

The New Atkins Diet is the more sustainable version of the infamous high-protein plan that limits carb intake, and that is the diet covered here.

The weight-loss promise

"Forget counting calories. Watch the fat melt away as a healthier and firmer body emerges. Enjoy more energy as well as freedom from a range of ailments, from diabetes to heart disease."

Dr Robert Atkins

The Atkins Diet is a low-carbohydrate, high-protein, weight-loss diet that was originally developed by Robert C. Atkins, M.D. in the 1960s. It has always been considered controversial because it originally allowed high-fat foods such as red meat, butter and cream, while banning foods seen as nutritious like wholemeal bread.

The diet's popularity has waxed and waned over the years, but in the early 1990s, Dr Atkins revived interest in his plan with the publication of his best-selling book *Dr. Atkins' New Diet Revolution*, which picked up a hefty celebrity following. Suddenly, it seemed as if everyone was on the Atkins Diet. In fact, it's now estimated that an incredible 20 million people worldwide have tried this particular diet.

However, one of the biggest criticisms of the Atkins Diet remained, namely that it was difficult to maintain eating so few carbohydrates over a long period of time. Robert Atkins died in 2003, but three other doctors took up the challenge of making Atkins more sustainable. Doctors Eric Westman, Stephen Phinney and Jeff Volek published *New Atkins, New*

You in 2010, promising "all the benefits of the original Atkins Diet in an improved, simplified form that can be tailored to your individual needs and sustained for the rest of your life".

The plan

You start on phase one, a low-carb diet designed for rapid weight loss, which lasts at least two weeks – depending on your weight-loss goal. During this phase, you're on three meals a day of protein, fat and very low-carbs, including meat, seafood, eggs, cheese, some veg, butter and oils. Phase one is designed to help you lose up to 15 lb (6.8 kg) in two weeks, reducing to 2–3 lb (900g–1.3 kg) a fortnight during the later phases. More carbs, fruit and veg are gradually introduced to your diet with the aim of working out what your "ideal carb intake" is to maintain a healthy weight for life.

While the old Atkins allowed you all the protein as you could eat, the New Atkins recommends 4–6 oz (115–175 g) with each meal, which is within healthy recommended amounts. There's no calorie counting, but some maths is involved because you have to be very exact about the amount of carbohydrates you consume. Vegetables are now allowed from day one – so much so that even vegetarians and vegans can follow this version of the diet. But you still mustn't eat sugar in any form (including in fruit juice) and the same goes for foods made from white flour or other refined grains, such as white bread, rice and pasta. Drinking two cups of coffee a day is encouraged, as it mildly enhances fat burning, but don't overdo it. Once the weight is off, you can slowly re-introduce carbohydrates – in a specific order, one at a time – to a maximum of 3½ oz (95 g) of carbs per day.

Exercise

Never a crucial part of old Atkins, exercise is gently encouraged under the new regime: "anything that gets you moving and elevates your heart rate" – walking, riding a bike, or even gardening for 20 minutes are all recommended.

How it works

Dr Atkins based his diet on the hypothesis that diets high in sugar and other refined carbohydrates increase the production of insulin, the hormone that stimulates the storage of calories as fat and can also lead to increased hunger and weight gain. So when you eat a high-carbohydrate meal, sugar from the carbohydrate quickly enters the bloodstream. To keep the blood sugar from rising too high, the body secretes insulin. Insulin allows the extra sugar to be stored in the liver and muscle as glycogen, but these stores are rapidly filled to capacity. The insulin then converts any extra sugar to fat.

The Atkins Diet severely restricts the consumption of carbohydrates, which as well as preventing the excess carbs from being stored as fat, also helps the body to burn the fat stores it already has. The body's primary source of energy is carbohydrates, but when you restrict the amount of carbohydrates you eat, it forces the body to metabolize fat to produce energy, a condition Atkins calls Benign Dietary Ketosis (BDK). The high-protein and fat levels in the diet are also supposed to keep you feeling pleasantly full and help control food cravings.

The initial fast-track phase of the New Atkins:

Breakfast	2 fried eggs, plus avocado with no-sugar salsa
Snack	Cucumber slices and 2 slices of Cheddar cheese
Lunch	Can of tuna, mixed green salad with cooked broccoli, spring onions, 4 pieces of marinated artichoke hearts and salad dressing
Snack	Roast turkey slices
Dinner	Burger (no bun) with 1 tablespoon of sautéed onions, 1 tablespoon of mushrooms, 2 slices Cheddar cheese and green salad with dressing

Who is it best for?

Lifestyle: You have a structured week, which requires that you are not to be disturbed by hunger pangs, but you have time to cook your own meals and keep a food diary.

Personality: Super-organized – you like to plan meals in advance and have no difficulty keeping track of what you've eaten.

PROS	CONS
• The diet can trigger rapid weight loss.	• The diet restricts important food groups, such as grains, fruits and dairy products.
• The high protein levels mean you won't feel hungry on this diet.	• It puts the body into a state of ketosis, which can cause a variety of unpleasant effects, such as headaches, bad breath and constipation.
• Today, there are more than 50 studies that highlight the positive weight-loss results and other health benefits associated with following the Atkins Diet, including reduction in risk for heart disease and diabetes.	• It's a fairly expensive diet to follow, as it involves eating a lot of meat.

Body shape: Apple – people who store fat around the middle are prone to high blood sugar, so need to watch their carb intake.

Any health concerns?

Many scientists voiced concerns about the old diet's long-term effect on cholesterol and the fact that the high intake of saturated fat may increase the risk of heart disease. New Atkins has tried to address this by recommending proteins lower in saturated fat than in the original plan, and some of the most recent research into low-carb diets suggests that they may actually have a positive effect on blood cholesterol.

However, most experts do agree that people with kidney problems shouldn't follow high-protein diets. Also, the restrictive nature of the initial phases of the plan can mean you miss out on some vital nutrients, and for this reason it's not suitable for pregnant or breastfeeding women, athletes and children. Starchy foods do make a huge contribution to vitamin and mineral intakes, such as B vitamins, calcium and iron, so cutting them out leaves you with potential gaps in your intake. A lack of fibre is also not beneficial for gut health.

It's also worth noting that many people on the diet don't generally reach the five-a-day portions of fruit and vegetable that are recommended to reduce heart disease, stroke and certain cancers.

Want to know more?

Read: *New Atkins, New You* by Dr Eric Westman, Dr Stephen Phinney and Dr Jeff Volek (Vermilion, 2010).

The Blood Type Diet

A bespoke diet plan based on your blood type.

The weight-loss promise:
"An individualized diet solution to staying healthy, living longer and achieving your ideal weight. Follow a menu and exercise plan that's carefully created to suit your blood type and, yes, you will shed those pounds."

Dr D'Adamo

This unique diet plan was first created more than 60 years ago by Dr James L. D'Adamo, a US doctor who believed that our blood types could directly affect our health and fitness. He was the first person to suggest that the types of food and exercise that each of us was best suited to depended on our blood type. His concept and the diet based on it have attracted many fans in the celebrity world but they have also come under immense fire from doctors and nutritionists for not being based on sound science.

Several books have been written since the original *Blood Type Diet*, including the most recent update by D'Adamo's son, Peter, called *Eat Right 4 Your Type*. "I've treated thousands of patients who've tried every weight-loss diet going and their single greatest complaint is that after all those months of dieting they just end up gaining the weight back," Dr D'Adamo Jnr explains. "I've discovered that in 95 per cent of my patients who struggle with their weight, it's down to eating the wrong foods for their blood type."

The plan

Eat Right 4 Your Type provides blood-type-specific diets to help you learn how to combine the foods that are right for you. Blood group O is the oldest blood group, so people with this type are told to follow a "hunter"-type diet like our ancient ancestors. This means high protein and avoiding too many carbs. Dairy should also be limited.

Blood group A evolved later than O, when people farmed more than they hunted, which apparently means they need less protein and more grains. In practice, this means eating less meat and lots more veg and wholemeal carbs.

Blood group B is recommended to eat vegetables and grains in a more balanced way – a bit of everything, basically, as lucky type Bs apparently lose weight easier than the rest of us.

Blood group AB is the newest and rarest blood type, apparently, so can digest a modern diet most easily. However, people those with this blood group are still advised to avoid too much meat and to pack the diet with mostly veggie foods.

Exercise

Dr D'Adamo believes your blood type also dictates the kind of exercise you should take. For example, he claims that people with Blood group O are very active and benefit from running, while those with A are more sedate and should work out less.

How it works

The elder D'Adamo says our blood type reflects our internal chemistry and determines the way we absorb nutrients. He believes that different blood types absorb certain foods better than others and handle stress differently – all of which, he

Blood group O

Breakfast	2 slices toasted spelt bread, ½ grapefruit, 1 poached egg, herbal tea, glass of water with lemon
Lunch	Turkey salad with lemon and olive oil dressing, 1 slice of wholegrain bread
Dinner	Lean grilled (broiled) steak, steamed broccoli, asparagus, peas and herbal tea
Exercise	Os are recommended to do a full hour of cardio, such as jogging, cycling, swimming or brisk walking, every day, preferably in the morning

Blood group A

Breakfast	Porridge with soya milk, herbal tea, glass of water with lemon
Lunch	Mixed green salad with hard-boiled eggs, herbal tea
Dinner	Salmon steak, steamed broccoli and kale, grilled tomatoes, herbal tea
Exercise	Apparently As are naturally less active than Os and need only 30 minutes' gentle exercise a day, such as yoga, thai chi or walking

Blood group B

Breakfast	Scrambled eggs on toast, glass of water with lemon, coffee
Lunch	Turkey breast and rice salad with veggies, herbal tea
Dinner	Steamed fish with steamed vegetables, fresh fruit
Exercise	Moderate exercise, especially team sports such as netball or dancing classes, two to three times a week for 30 minutes

Blood group AB

Breakfast	Grapefruit juice, 2 slices of toast, poached egg, glass of water with lemon
Lunch	Turkey breast on rye bread, Caesar salad, herbal tea
Dinner	Cheese omelette, stir-fried vegetables, mixed-fruit salad
Exercise	Mix it up with gentle yoga or Pilates once a week and a couple of sessions of something more intense, such as light jogging

PROS	CONS
• Recommends eating fresh, natural foods and cutting out convenience meals, alcohol, chocolate and coffee.	• There is no solid scientific evidence to back up the theory that your blood type has any bearing on your digestion.
• You'll probably lose weight because, regardless of your blood type, it's a very restricted diet.	• You'll need a blood test to discover your blood group if you don't already know it.

claims, plays a key role in losing weight and avoiding disease. The theory supporting this claim is that because each blood type evolved at a different point in history, we should adopt diets similar to the ones our ancestors had when the blood group first evolved. Dr D'Adamo claims that by eating the foods that your blood type can easily digest, you will lose weight, feel healthier and live for longer.

Who is it best for?

Lifestyle: You have lots of time to think about food, cooking and shopping.

Personality: You're looking for a new approach to dieting and like the thought of an individualized plan – and have the conviction to make a permanent change.

Body shape: Any – the idea is that the diet suits your blood type, regardless of your body shape.

Any health concerns?

Most medical experts say there is no established link between our blood group and how we process food, and therefore you won't find qualified dieticians recommending this plan. Another concern is that some of the plans, especially those recommended for blood groups O and A, are considerably limited and cut out major food groups altogether. In the long term, this can result in a poor intake of the nutrients needed for good health. Cutting out dairy products, for example, will lead to a lower intake of iodine, riboflavin and calcium, which can put women at a higher risk of the bone-thinning condition osteoporosis, while avoiding meat can result in low levels of iron, which can lead to anaemia.

Want to know more?

Read: *Eat Right 4 Your Type* by Dr Peter D'Adamo with Catherine Whitney (Century, 1998).

Cabbage Soup Diet

Based on guzzling vegetable soup and little else, a classic crash diet with all the corresponding health risks.

The weight-loss promise:
Lose 10–15 lb (4.5–6.8 kg) in seven days.

Rumours surround the origin of this quick-fix plan, but no one has ever stepped forward claiming to be its creator! Instructions for the Cabbage Soup Diet began doing the rounds in the 1980s, when they went viral via fax machines and word of mouth. However, the diet appears to have no links to a book, doctor, nutritionist or other expert source. This inevitably led to speculation, and the diet was linked to a wide variety of sources, including the US military and the Sacred Heart Memorial Hospital, which prompted the hospital to issue a statement saying that it had not created the diet and did not consider it a healthy way of controlling weight. Due to its unknown origins, a Chinese whispers-effect occurred among followers, which has led to multiple variations of the diet and the cabbage soup recipe around which it centres.

The plan

All versions of the diet have a strict list of what to eat each day for a week. The diet is based around cabbage soup, with a few other low-calorie foods, such as fruit, vegetables, skimmed milk and meat, to supplement it. There is no limit on how much cabbage soup can be consumed on any given day. The plan also encourages drinking plenty of water and avoiding alcohol. Due to the extreme low-calorie and low-protein content of this diet, it is only ever advised that you follow it for a week at a time.

The cabbage soup recipe varies slightly among different versions of the diet, but it basically includes cabbage and assorted low-calorie vegetables such as onions, celery, carrots, peppers, mushrooms and tomatoes, and is most often flavoured with stock and tomato juice. There is no exercise plan to accompany the diet.

How it works

The diet makes no fancy scientific claims as to how it works. There's nothing magical about cabbage or cabbage soup that triggers weight loss, but even those with big appetites will only be able to eat so much of the soup every day, so the reason this diet seems to work is because you don't consume many calories! The Cabbage Soup Diet is essentially a modified fast, containing so few calories that dieters lose a lot of weight rapidly. However, most of the initial weight loss will primarily be from fluids rather than fat, and the weight will therefore return once the dieter resumes eating normally.

Who is it best for?

Lifestyle: You only cook for yourself (not for a family). A balanced diet isn't something that usually features high on your priority list and you've left it to the last minute to get in shape for an upcoming special event or holiday.

Personality: You're task-focused, like to see results quickly and you don't want to be tied down to any sort of regime for longer than a week.

The idea is to eat as much cabbage soup as you like every day – enough to keep you full up – plus specific additional foods on each day of the week.

Day 1	Unlimited cabbage soup and fruit (excluding bananas). Water to drink
Day 2	Cabbage soup and additional vegetables. 1 jacket potato with butter for dinner. No fruit
Day 3	Unlimited cabbage soup plus any fruit and vegetables you choose (excluding potatoes or bananas)
Day 4	Unlimited cabbage soup and skimmed milk, plus bananas
Day 5	Unlimited cabbage soup, 1 lb 5 oz (600 g) beef and 6 tomatoes. Drink 6–8 glasses of water to flush extra uric acid from your body
Day 6	Unlimited cabbage soup and limitless beef and vegetables (excluding potatoes)
Day 7	Unlimited cabbage soup with a little brown rice, vegetables and water

PROS	CONS
• It's easy to follow, as there's no calorie or carb counting and no recommended exercise regime or lifestyle changes to make.	• If you lose a lot of weight very quickly, it's unlikely that you're actually losing much fat – just water weight.
• You will lose weight rapidly, and the limited nature of the diet means that it's cheap to follow.	• As you won't be making any lasting changes to your eating habits, you will probably quickly regain any weight lost.
• It only lasts for a week.	• The large amounts of cabbage can cause wind.
	• The restrictive nature of the diet means it's very boring.
	• Despite being allowed limitless bowls of soup, you will probably still feel constantly hungry.

Body shape: Large: this diet involves no exercise – and on such a low-calorie allowance you'll struggle to have the energy to do any – so if your aim is to target and tone up problem areas, it probably won't help you.

Any health concerns?

Followed for only a week, the Cabbage Soup Diet does not last long enough to severely harm healthy individuals, but the extreme plan has some worrying aspects nonetheless. The theory is comparable to very low-calorie diets used to treat clinical obesity. However, these plans, administered by professionals, typically use fortified meal replacements with added nutrients. Experts agree that any diet under 1,200 calories per day is unsafe unless it is medically supervised.

Apart from high amounts of salt, the ingredients of the cabbage soup are in themselves mostly healthy – however, it's almost impossible to get all the nutrients you need and properly satisfy hunger with so few calories. The cabbage diet is unsurprisingly deficient in protein, carbohydrate and essential fats ,and if you were to follow it long term, it would result in severe nutritional deficiencies.

If you have an underlying health condition, the potential adverse side effects of even a week could be more serious. For example, a diabetic could struggle to keep glucose levels under control. In short, the medical consensus is that it's a fad crash diet and best avoided.

Want to know more?

Visit: www.cabbage-soup-diet.com

The Cambridge Diet

Replace solid food with liquid shakes and watch the pounds fall off.

The weight-loss promise:
It's safe, convenient, easy-to-use and nutritionally balanced, and offers flexible diet programmes that give real results.

The Cambridge Diet is the original "meal replacement" weight-loss plan. Developed in the 1960s at Cambridge University by Dr Alan Howard, the diet was launched commercially in the US in 1980 and in the UK in 1984. Now known as the Cambridge Weight Plan, it's a liquid-based diet, originally intended for morbidly obese patients and based on the Very Low Calorie Diet (VLCD) model. In essence, it replaces food with nutritionally complete but low-calorie shakes, soups and meal-replacement bars. The meal replacement lasts until the person meets his or her weight-loss goal. In the UK, you need to meet with a trained Cambridge Diet advisor before starting the diet. Having been around for more than 40 years, the plan has stood the test of time and still has a loyal following today, although its critics say it is too extreme and may trigger health problems.

The plan

The Cambridge Weight Plan is based around buying the range of meal-replacement products and following one of its six flexible diet plans, with increasing daily calorie amounts, depending on your starting weight. There is also a long-term weight-management programme to help you keep slim once the weight is off. The bars, soups, porridges and shakes can be used as your sole source of nutrition or together with low-calorie regular meals, again depending on your starting size. While on the programme, you receive advice and support from a Cambridge adviser and buy your products from them. They advise which step is the most appropriate for you to start on, calculated by your current weight and how active you are.

Depending on how much weight you need to lose, the daily calorie allowance can vary from between 440 and 1,500 calories, and a plan can be either all meal-replacement products or a mixture of products and normal foods. For example, on Step 1, you will consume three or four meal-replacement products a day and no "real" food, totalling around 440 calories per day. But by the time you reach Step 5, you're allowed 1,500 calories per day, which typically consists of one diet product and a normal but healthy breakfast, dinner, lunch and snack.

Exercise

You should not exercise during Step 1, as the calorie intake is so low, but moderate exercise is encouraged during the later steps of the plan.

How it works

Like all VLCDs, the Cambridge initially works by forcing your body into ketosis – a state in which you are undernourished and your body must process your fat stores in order to survive. This is just a temporary stage. After this, weight loss is down to the simple fact that you consume far fewer calories. The idea behind meal replacements is that they contain all the essential nutrients you need in fewer calories, so allow people to lose weight without having to think about food. The replacement process is designed to take away the need to make any food decisions by removing you from situations such as shopping, cooking, mealtimes and eating out. As a result, your calorie intake is carefully controlled and you lose weight.

Who is it best for?

Lifestyle: You're too busy to plan your own meals or perhaps you don't fancy the extra cooking that comes with most plans.

Personality: You struggle with self-control or low motivation and would benefit from someone else taking charge of the situation and telling you what to eat and when.

Body shape: Obese or very overweight. Meal-replacement diets can be very effective if you have a serious weight problem and have tried and failed to lose weight using traditional diets.

Any health concerns?

Extreme calorie restriction is a constant source of controversy. Diets based on severe calorie restriction, as in the first steps of this diet, have been proven to work, especially for the very overweight, but if they're not carefully monitored they can also result in side effects, including light-headedness and fainting, nausea, irritability, diarrhoea, muscle loss, temporary hair loss and constipation.

As a result, the UK's National Obesity Forum suggests that very low calorie diets (VLCDs) should be used only under close medical and dietetic supervision, and recommends people are

PROS	CONS
• It can work when all else has failed – many people find the weight-loss results quite dramatic after years of struggling on other diets.	• Cost – buying the meal-replacement products every week can work out quite expensive.
• The meal replacements are all nutritionally balanced, so you're likely to be getting all the vitamins and minerals you need, albeit not from real food.	• Initial side effects can include bad breath, a dry mouth, tiredness, dizziness, insomnia, nausea and constipation from cutting down on carbs and fibre.
• There's a coach on hand to provide encouragement and advice.	• Repeated weight loss and regain – otherwise known as yo-yo dieting – is a big risk with meal-replacement diets. After following the plan, some people simply return to their previous lifestyle and so the weight comes straight back on.
	• Sticking to it. Giving up normal meals and swapping them for a snack bar or a shake can be boring and feel socially isolating. This isn't a plan you can stick to in the long term.
	• Your advisor is ultimately there to sell you products.

medically assessed before starting one and are then closely monitored throughout the treatment. It's important that you have support from your doctor if you're following the very low calorie phase of the plan, and that you don't try to exercise while consuming too few daily calories.

Probably the most common serious side effect seen with VLCDs is gallstone formation. These painful stones frequently develop in obese people and are even more common during rapid weight loss. The reason for this may be that restricting food intake decreases the gallbladder's ability to empty out bile, causing hard stones to form.

Meal replacement programmes may not help establish a new healthy eating pattern that can be maintained long term.

Want to know more?

Visit: www.cambridgeweightplan.com

The Clean and Lean Diet

Ditch the junk from your diet and get a body like "The Body".

The weight-loss promise:
To achieve your "maximum individual genetic potential" and get the body you've always wanted – with no calorie counting or complicated rules.

Almost 20 years ago, James Duigan moved from Adelaide to London to study fitness and personal training. He met Elle Macpherson four years later when she approached him at the gym where he was working and asked if he would train her. "We worked on my body, attitude, balance, strength and consistency," Macpherson writes in her foreword to Duigan's bestselling book *Clean & Lean Diet*, describing her workouts. "James's approach is non-gimmicky and straightforward. Soon I got in the best shape ever – mentally and physically."

Duigan has since worked with a host of other celebrities and also launched his own company, Bodyism, an exclusive gym in London's Kensington. He's also gone on to publish other books based on his "clean food" approach.

The plan

The Clean and Lean programme takes the form of a 14-day Kick-start Plan, which consists of three meals plus snacks every day, all of which primarily contain vegetables and protein such as poultry, fish and eggs, and very little – if any – carbs. The aim is to cut out anything that's toxic to the body. The main culprits according to James are what he defines as C.R.A.P: caffeine, refined sugar, alcohol and processed foods. Wheat and wheat products such as breads, pasta and cereal must also be limited. You are allowed one cheat meal a week because you will be eating correctly for the rest of the week.

The diet is made up of "clean" foods that haven't changed much from their natural state (for example, a crisp looks nothing like a potato, but a baked spud is fine), don't require any added flavourings, don't last for months and contain preservatives, don't contain more than five or six ingredients, don't contain ingredients that you can't pronounce or that you don't recognize, and don't list sugar as one of the first three ingredients.

You should eat good fat every day – the heart-friendly kind found in nuts, avocados, oily fish and oils. Fruit is banned for the first two weeks due to its high sugar content but you should drink 2–3 litres of still, filtered (not tap) water a day – and you're allowed one cup of organic coffee or tea. Probiotics and prebiotics are also included in the diet, either in foods that contain them or supplements.

Chewing each mouthful properly is encouraged – it should take at least 20 minutes to finish a meal. After the Kick-start Plan, the aim is to adopt a sensible eating regime that consists of "clean" foods.

Exercise

Throughout the plan, dieters have to complete an 8-minute workout every day and, if they have time, follow that with a 20-minute walk.

How it works

Duigan's diet is founded on the principle that lean is the body's natural state. He believes the body doesn't naturally cling onto fat – it's only when you eat processed foods and drinks and your body becomes full of toxins that fat sticks. In his view, the fat clings to these toxins. So far, the scientific evidence to back up these central claims is thin, but Duigan is convinced that the body stores toxins in fat cells, and unless you clear out the toxins you'll find it hard to keep the pounds off. Toxins, including caffeine, refined sugar and alcohol, are apparently the reason most diets are a waste of time. If you go on a diet yet still eat the wrong toxin-filled foods, such as low-fat treats and diet soft drinks, you may lose weight at first, but the toxins

DAILY MENU EXAMPLE	
Breakfast	A glass of water with a squeeze of lemon or lime, scrambled egg, 1¾ oz (50 g) smoked salmon and a cup of spinach
Snack	6 nuts
Lunch	Spinach omelette (2 eggs) with a slice of turkey or smoked salmon and green salad
Snack	Chopped veg and 1 tablespoon of houmous
Dinner	Lamb kebabs with cooked spiced beetroot, spinach, broccoli and peppers

PROS	CONS
• The initial phase is short – just two weeks.	• Shopping for clean foods with short shelf lives is time-consuming. You'll need extra time to follow the diet religiously.
• The 8-minute exercises are easy to fit in to your daily routine and can be done at home, so there's no costly gym membership required.	• Drinking only bottled water and eating fresh organic foods is expensive.
• You are allowed "cheat" meals, so no need to panic if you fall off the wagon.	• This diet is designed for carnivores – not good news if you're a vegetarian.

have nowhere to go other than back into your system. This is why you often feel tired, lethargic and headachy soon after starting a diet, he says. Your body reacts by holding on to fat in order to store the toxins. So if you're toxic, goes the theory, you'll always struggle to lose weight, but if you stick to clean foods that are toxin-free, unprocessed and close to their natural state, you should lose weight easily and keep it off.

Who is it best for?

Lifestyle: You're meticulously tidy and spend a lot of time making sure everything from your home to your hair is in tiptop condition. The "clean" philosophy of this plan will tally with your own personal philosophy of life. It also helps if you're into alternative medicine and believe that science doesn't always know all the answers.

Personality: You're a follower – you may have difficulty creating plans for yourself, but love following set diet plans and will enjoy the challenge of working with lists of permitted and banned foods.

Body shape: Pot-bellied – stress can cause storage of fat around the middle. Duigan believes a diet full of toxins puts stress on the body, so by eliminating them from your diet you'll notice your stomach becoming flatter.

Any health concerns?

Overall this is a pretty healthy diet, which only restricts unhealthy processed or "junk" foods and is packed with whole grains, vegetables and lean protein. On the other hand, banning fruit – which is packed with vitamins and disease-fighting antioxidants – even just for the first two weeks of the plan isn't a good health strategy.

Also, bear in mind that there is also absolutely no robust science to back up Duigan's theory that "fat clings on to toxins" and by eating his "clean" foods you'll lose weight faster. You will lose weight on the diet, but mainly because you'll be cutting down on calories overall, as it eliminates high-calorie junk food. Another possible downside is that because the regime is so strict about ditching naughty food, there's a good chance you'll fall off the wagon or simply return to old diet habits once the plan is over.

Want to know more?

Read: *Clean & Lean Diet* by James Duigan (Kyle Books, 2012).

Detox

A family of restrictive diets that believes eating mainly fruit and veg flushes out toxins – and fat along with them.

The weight-loss promise:
Detox diets claim to flush poisons from your body, purge pounds of excess fat, improve digestion, clear your complexion, strengthen hair and nails, bolster the immune system; banish cellulite and leave you feeling energized.

The premise of detoxing is based on the ancient Greek belief that we need to periodically clear the "toxic waste" from our body in order to stay healthy. Originally, detoxing also had a spiritual element, and fasting, which is part of many detox diets, is still practised by people of many faiths.

In recent years, this idea of cleansing the body has become popular again; the word "detox" has become a buzzword in the world of health products, and been attached to a variety of different diets plans. There are now a vast number of detox plans, from juice diets to everyday cleanses to lemon detox, many of them endorsed by celebrities. One such plan is the Master Cleanse, which encourages you to ingest only a mixture of water, lemons, cayenne pepper and maple syrup up to six times a day for 10 days. However, medical experts warn that extreme detox diets such as this can be very dangerous.

The plan

The many detox diet books and kits on the market each have their own take on how to cleanse the body – one calls for spices, another for only vegetable purées – but most of them boil down to very low-calorie, basically liquid diets. Detox diets can last from around one day to about a month. They all centre on cutting out certain elements of your diet, such as processed foods, and consuming an extremely limited list of foods instead – for example, only fruit and veg. Detox diets are often high in fibre to help flush out the system and may also involve total fasting for short periods of time. Other common rules include avoiding caffeine and alcohol and eliminating potential dietary allergens such as wheat and dairy. Some detox diets recommend using herbs and other supplements, along with enemas, to cleanse the intestines.

Most detox diets follow three basic steps: First, they aim to flush all waste from your body with a very restricted diet, then they reintroduce plant-based foods and, lastly, they broaden out to include a larger variety of still very healthy foods.

Exercise

Most plans don't involve much exercise, apart from a bit of yoga, as consuming so few calories means you won't have the energy.

How it works

Detoxing is based on the concept that your body needs help to get rid of unwanted "toxins" – accumulated harmful substances that are alleged to exert undesirable effects on health, including the storage of excess fat. Of course, our bodies have their own in-built detoxification system that includes our kidneys, liver and even our skin. However, detox advocates believe that the current burden of toxins in our modern food and environment is too much for our evolutionary system to handle and so these toxins build up leading to problems such as weight gain, cellulite, headaches and bad

DAILY MENU EXAMPLE	
On waking	Warm water with a squeeze of lemon
Breakfast	Porridge made with almond milk and berries, herbal tea
Snack	Apple and a handful of almonds
Lunch	Vegetable soup topped with toasted pumpkin seeds (no bread)
Snack	Carrot sticks with homemade houmous
Dinner	Steamed fish with veggies

skin. Current scientific evidence to support this theory is thin but the argument runs that once free of toxins, your body functions better and your metabolism works super-efficiently, helping you shed those extra pounds.

Who are they best for?

Lifestyle: You go through phases of overindulging a little, for example at Christmas or during busy periods at work, but between these times you have breaks from socializing and work commitments when you can focus on your health.

PROS	CONS
• The plans don't last too long and you will see quick results, which can boost self-confidence.	• They are quite monotonous and need a lot of willpower to stick to.
• It's common to experience fewer cravings for sugar and caffeine, and to feel satisfied with smaller portions of food.	• Those that severely limit protein or require fasting can result in fatigue.
• Detox diets encourage some good habits, such as eating more fruit and vegetables, drinking more water and cutting down on caffeine, alcohol and junk food. They also help you to think about what you're eating.	• They can be short on many nutrients, leading to certain deficiencies and lowered immunity.
	• They often involve buying juice or supplements, which can be expensive, and they can make socializing difficult, as few restaurants and bars will cater for your diet.
	• Much of the weight lost initially will be water and will be quickly regained once the detox is over.

Personality: You're very focused, you don't get bored easily and you crave structure. You are extremely determined, don't give up easily and always see a plan through to its end.

Body shape: Bloated – for those who suffer from bloating, the high-fibre nature of detox diets might help soothe the digestive system.

Any health concerns?

Many doctors dispute the need for detox diets, claiming that there is no scientific evidence that they work, and that in fact the body is perfectly capable of clearing out harmful substances by itself.

When you starve your body of calories, your body starts to release chemicals called ketones, which can trigger nausea, dehydration, light-headedness and irritability. Plus a prolonged lack of protein causes your body to break down its own muscles and can compromise your immune system. Foods such as wheat and dairy, which are often cut out on detoxes, are a source of important nutrients, so it's potentially harmful to exclude them from the diet. People who suspect they have a true allergy to dairy or wheat should be diagnosed by a qualified doctor and should not self-diagnose.

It does make sense to avoid excessive intakes of caffeine, alcohol and high-fat, high-sugar foods. However, a detox is an extreme way to go about this and impossible to keep up long term. A better long-term approach is to stick to the recommended balanced diet that includes five portions of different fruit and veg a day, plenty of wholegrain cereals, lean meat, fish and low-fat dairy.

You should always check with your doctor before you start any diet, especially one as extreme as a detox plan, because they can cause further health problems for people with pre-existing conditions, such as diabetes, and can be dangerous if you're pregnant or breastfeeding.

Want to know more?

Read: *Detox Yourself: Feel the Difference in 7 Days* by Jane Scrivner (Piatkus, 2007).

The Dukan Diet

The French high-protein answer to the Atkins that allows you to enjoy meals out while you slim.

The weight-loss promise:
"A unique 4-step programme, combining two steps to lose your unwanted weight and two steps to keep it off for good."

Dr Dukan

Designed by French doctor Pierre Dukan, this diet claims you can lose 10 lb (4.5 kg) in just five days and is credited with helping over four million women in his home country shed their unwanted flab. But the plan only really captured international attention when it was reported in the press that Carole Middleton – mother of Prince William's wife, Kate Middleton – followed Dr Dukan's high-protein diet to ensure that her figure was slim for the Royal Wedding in April 2011.

French medic Dr Pierre Dukan first created his protein-based diet in the 1970s, when an obese patient asked for a diet plan that would really work for a change. The patient's only caveat was that he had to be allowed to eat meat. Dr Dukan told the man to eat nothing but protein and drink plenty of water – then come back in a week. When the patient returned, just five days later, a full 10 lb (4.5 kg) lighter, Dukan knew that he'd hit on something.

But following its soaring success, there came criticism from some quarters that the diet was not healthy and, after a falling out with the medical community, Dr Dukan ceased to be a member of the *Ordre des médecins* – the official French medical board.

The plan

Dukan is a low-carbohydrate, high-protein diet. There's no limit to how much you can eat during the plan's four phases, provided you stick to the rules of the plan. Dukan recommends you take a multi-vitamin while following it, to ensure you don't miss out on important nutrients. He also advises drinking plenty of water and consuming 1–3 tablespoons of oat bran daily, to combat constipation and hunger pangs.

1. The Attack Phase
To kick-start the diet, you eat just protein for 2–7 days – only lean meat, fish, eggs and non-fat dairy foods are suggested. Strenuous activity is to be avoided during this phase.

2. The Cruise Phase
Carry on as above, but add in unlimited non-starchy veg every other day. This "on and off" diet continues until you reach your target weight.

3. The Consolidation Phase
Once at your ideal weight, you can re-introduce foods such as bread, pasta, rice, butter and vegetable oils. During this stage you're not expected to lose weight but simply to maintain your target weight. A weekly "celebration" of a main course, dessert and glass of wine is allowed.

4. The Stabilization Phase
You can eat whatever you like for six days a week, but stick to three basic rules: eat only protein on Thursdays for the rest of your life, walk 20 minutes a day and consume three tablespoons of oat bran a day.

During the Attack phase

Breakfast	A fat-free yogurt or fromage frais, and a boiled egg with 1 slice of turkey or lean ham
Lunch	Oat bran pancake with salmon or fat-free cottage cheese
Dinner	Grilled (broiled) fish or chicken breast cooked with lemon juice and paprika

Exercise

Walking for 20–30 minutes each day is recommended.

How it works

This is a high-protein diet that, according to Dukan, works because, ounce for ounce, proteins are relatively low in calories when compared to fats and carbs, plus their complex structure means they're pretty hard work for the body to digest. As a result, you burn up more calories processing proteins than any other food, which, he claims, makes weight loss inevitable and swift.

According to Dukan, the reason why many diets fail in the long term and people end up putting all the weight back on is because eating too little impairs your body's metabolism. "It's a survival tactic," he says. "If you skip meals, the next time you

PROS	CONS
• You tend to lose weight quickly, which is motivating.	• It's actually stricter than the Atkins diet in the first phases and almost impossible to follow if you're vegetarian.
• You don't need to weigh food or count calories. Apart from keeping to low-fat, low-salt and high-protein foods, there's no restriction on how much you can eat during your first two weeks.	• At the start of the diet you may experience side effects, such as bad breath, a dry mouth, tiredness, dizziness, insomnia and nausea, from cutting out carbs.
• You can still eat out if you pick a simple meat or fish dish and skip dessert.	• The lack of whole grains, fruit and veg in the early stages of the diet could cause constipation.
	• There's no mention of portion sizes and, ultimately to lose weight, you need to eat fewer calories than you burn.
	• Only eating protein on a Thursday permanently will mean eating out on this day is tricky – for ever.

eat, your body will become a sponge and absorb 100 per cent of calories instead of 70." To combat this, the final stage of his diet provides a transition between strict dieting and a return to normal eating, which, he says, will keep you slim for life.

Who is it best for?

Lifestyle: You're busy, sociable and eat out a lot. You also want results quickly.

Personality: People who like rules. It's a very strict and prescriptive diet, which some people like. Naturally, it also suits happy carnivores who can think of little better than a juicy steak.

Body shape: Pot bellied – as a low-carb diet, there is some evidence that reducing carbs can help shift belly fat.

Any health concerns?

In 2012 the British Dietetic Association named Dukan the worst celeb diet plan of the year. Why? Well, it's not a nutritionally balanced diet and doesn't follow the general healthy eating guidelines that research has established help keep us healthy. For example, in the first phases you may miss out on key nutrients, such as calcium and vitamin D, and disease-fighting antioxidants from fruits and whole grains. Plus there is a lack of variety of fibre-rich foods. Having oat bran every day is also not something that most health experts would recommend. Oat bran contains phytates, naturally occurring compounds that can bind with minerals such as iron and zinc and reduce their absorption, so there are healthy ways to get more fibre – such as eating plenty of fruit and veg.

Want to know more?

Read: *The Dukan Diet* by Dr Pierre Dukan (Hodder, 2010).

The GI Diet

Swap white carbs for brown, and avoid sugar altogether – simple!

The weight-loss promise:
"In theory you can lose up to 10 lb in a month. But I recommend losing weight more slowly – say, around a pound a week. Apart from helping you to lose weight, this diet helps prevent heart disease and strokes."

Rick Gallop

Before 1994, all patients diagnosed with diabetes were instructed to avoid sugary foods because they were known to cause a rapid rise in blood glucose levels. At the same time, they were told not to worry about eating carbohydrates such as bread, because these were thought to release glucose more slowly into the blood and, therefore, not interfere with blood glucose control. And yet, even when patients carefully followed this advice, their blood sugar wasn't always kept under control.

David Jenkins, a professor of nutrition at the University of Toronto, Canada, decided to find out why. During a series of tests, he discovered that eating the carbohydrates in white bread elevated a subject's blood glucose more than eating sugary ice cream. Scientists subsequently tested all carbohydrate foods and compiled the glycaemic index (GI) table, which outlines how different carbs affect blood glucose levels – an impact that can vary enormously.

The GI table was later used to develop a successful line of diet books, based on eating foods with a low GI, authored by Rick Gallop, former president of the Heart and Stroke

Foundation of Ontario. Gallop's first book on the subject, *GI Diet*, published in 2003, transformed the glycaemic index theory into an easy weight-loss diet. It appeared on *The New York Times* bestseller list and has sold over two million copies. Since then, a number of different GI diets have been devised.

The plan

You must eat only carbs with a low GI, such as brown bread and wholewheat pasta, and avoid those with a high GI, including potatoes, white rice, white flour, refined grains and sugary foods like chocolate. In Gallop's version of the diet, foods are grouped into three coloured categories. Foods from the "red" group have a high GI and should be avoided; foods from the "yellow" group can be eaten in moderation; and foods from the "green" group have a low GI and can be eaten without limitation. The eating plan also promotes a healthy ratio between carbohydrates, lean proteins and healthy fats. The golden rule is: don't go hungry – your digestive system must be kept active. This means no more than three hours between meals and snacks.

The diet kicks off with an introductory weight-loss phase in which pulses and grains are excluded, followed by a less severe maintenance diet. You're encouraged to have healthy treats such as homemade apple muffins, low-fat ice cream and even dark chocolate. Caffeine should be avoided, as it stimulates appetite, while alcohol is discouraged because it has a high GI.

Exercise

You're not expected to exercise during phase one of the diet, but during phase two, 30 minutes of activity per day is recommended to accelerate weight loss.

How it works

A low-GI diet is a weight-loss diet based on controlling blood sugar. The glycaemic index measures the speed at which carbohydrates break down in the digestive system to form glucose (sugar), the body's source of energy. Glucose is set at 100 and all carbohydrates are indexed against that number, on a scale of 0 to 100, based on their impact on blood glucose levels after eating. Foods that are digested quickly have a high GI, and foods that are digested more slowly have a lower GI. Peanut butter, for example, has a low GI of 14, while cornflakes raise blood sugar levels very quickly and so have a GI score of 92.

When you eat high-GI foods, your body rapidly converts the carbs into glucose, which dissolves in your blood stream, spiking your blood sugar level and giving you a sugar rush. This sugar spike is short-lived because insulin takes this sugar from the bloodstream and stores it for immediate use in your muscles – with the excess stored as fat around your waist, hips and thighs. The higher the spike, the higher the level of insulin released and the quicker the sugar is drained from your bloodstream, leaving you with a sugar low – which inevitably leads you to look for a sugar fix. In summary – a diet of high-GI foods makes you feel hungry more often, which means you end up eating more and putting on weight.

The principle of the GI diet maintains that the best way to keep hunger at bay while consuming fewer calories is to eat low-GI foods that deliver glucose to the bloodstream at a slow and steady rate.

Who is it best for?

Lifestyle: You are busy and can't afford to feel hungry,

From phase 1

Breakfast	Porridge made with skimmed milk
Snack	Oatcakes with low-fat houmous
Lunch	Grilled (broiled) salmon or chicken with new potatoes and asparagus or salad
Afternoon snack	Low-fat yogurt
Dinner	Lamb and bean stew with basmati rice, plus two squares of very dark chocolate

deprived or tired. You need to be able to eat nutritious food on the go and to pick up meals that won't ruin your plans when you're out and about.

Personality: You have a short attention span, bore easily and thrive on variety, so would be unable to stick to diets that ban foods. At the same time, you are patient enough to wait for modest results.

Body shape: Apple – people who store fat round the middle are more at risk of developing type 2 diabetes, so a diet that balances out insulin levels will be good for them.

PROS	CONS
• Switching from a high GI-index diet to a low-GI diet can be done relatively easily.	• It's difficult to work out the glycaemic load of a meal, as the preparation and combination of foods can alter their glycaemic index.
• This is no crash diet, and a moderate rate of weight loss is definitely beneficial for general health.	• It's unlikely that following the rules of the GI diet can help you lose a lot of body fat in a short space of time.
• No food group is banned, making this diet easy to stick to and ensuring you get a good range of nutrients.	

Any health concerns?

The glycaemic index doesn't take into account food nutrition content. Indeed, some foods with the preferred lower GI ranking may, in fact, be less healthy because they contain large amounts of calories, sugar or saturated fat, especially packaged and processed foods. For example, crisps (potato chips) and ice cream have a lower GI ranking than baked potatoes, even though baked potatoes are generally considered healthier. Brown and white rice rank comparably on the index scale, as do white and wholewheat bread, yet by most scientific measures the whole-grain choices are healthier. So while lower GI items may help balance blood sugar, choosing them indiscriminately could lead to other health problems.

Want to know more?

Read: *The GI Diet: The Glycemic Index – The Easy, Healthy Way to Permanent Weight Loss* by Rick Gallop (Virgin Books, 2005).

Gluten-Free

Ditch wheat and other glutinous grains to help banish both bloating and flab.

The weight-loss promise:
Alongside all the digestive health benefits, some gluten-free plans promise you'll drop up to 10 lb (4.5 kg) in just two weeks.

The gluten-free diet was originally developed to help combat coeliac disease – an autoimmune condition in which gluten, found in wheat, barley and rye, triggers an immune reaction that damages the lining of the small intestine. Coeliac disease affects around 1 in 100 people, and symptoms range from mild bloating and indigestion to more severe stomach pain, diarrhoea and anaemia, caused by a lack of iron because nutrients aren't properly absorbed. Gluten was first identified as a trigger for the disease in 1950, when Dutch paediatrician Willem Dicke found that removing wheat from the diet caused the symptoms to disappear. The gluten-free diet has transformed the lives of millions with the disease and is still the cornerstone of treatment today.

It wasn't until recent years that the diet started to be used for weight-loss purposes, with a range of high-profile celebs, including Gwyneth Paltrow, saying they avoid gluten. Host of American TV show *The View*, Elisabeth Hasselbeck, helped popularize the diet by publishing *The G-Free Diet* in 2009, after being diagnosed with coeliac disease herself. Although *The G-Free Diet* advises against self-diagnosis and encourages people to see a doctor for testing, it does promote a gluten-free diet for other reasons, including weight loss, controlling

IBS, increasing energy, improving attention span and speeding digestion. "Even people with no health issues have a great deal to gain by giving up gluten," Hasselbeck writes.

The plan

You cut out all grains that contain gluten, which means no wheat, rye and barley. The most obvious sources of gluten are wheat flour, breakfast cereals and anything made with wheat flour, including bread, pasta, pizza bases, cakes, pastries, biscuits (cookies), and anything coated in batter or breadcrumbs. Gluten can also be found in less obvious foods, such as soups, sauces, beer, ready (convenience) meals, processed foods such as sausages, and even some ice creams and crisps (potato chips). This is because thickeners and coatings used in these foods are often made from wheat. To make it easier to identify those foods containing gluten, any ingredient that's derived from wheat, barley, rye or oats has to be identified in the ingredients list on the packaging by law.

The gluten-free diet is made up of naturally gluten-free foods, such as meat, fish, fruit and vegetables, rice, potatoes, lentils, and certain grains like buckwheat, quinoa and millet. Processed foods that don't contain gluten and gluten-free substitute foods (available in most supermarkets), such as bread, flour, pasta, crackers and biscuits, are also available.

Exercise

There isn't a specific recommended exercise plan to go with a gluten-free diet plan. However, as carbs are a key source of fuel for people exercising, and carbs often contain wheat and other gluten sources, it's important to find gluten-free carbs to keep up your energy levels if you are working out.

DAILY MENU EXAMPLE	
Breakfast	Buckwheat pancakes with fresh berries and maple syrup
Lunch	Homemade ramen (rice) noodle soup with chicken and vegetables
Dinner	Gluten-free sausages with baked sweet potato, broccoli, courgette (zucchini) and peas
Snack	Apple, 8 Brazil nuts

How it works

The theory behind gluten-free weight-loss diets is that most people, even those without coeliac disease, can't fully digest gluten, lacking certain enzymes needed to break it down. Proponents believe that we'd all be better off not eating wheat and other gluten-containing grains. Some also claim that the reason wheat causes dietary problems is because it has been changed through modern farming practices and genetic modification, and is completely different from the "natural" wheat eaten by our ancestors.

Who is it best for?

Lifestyle: Food is at the heart of your daily life and you're a keen cook. If you already check labels and love tweaking recipes, creating gluten-free meals will be easy for you.

PROS	CONS
• If you have undiagnosed coeliac disease or a sensitivity to wheat, this diet could resolve your health problems.	• Lack of fibre in your diet from traditional sources can lead to digestive issues.
• Encourages label reading and more general awareness of foods.	• It's difficult to completely avoid all forms of gluten, as it hides in many sauces and condiments.
• To avoid gluten, you need to eat fewer processed foods.	• Simply choosing food products that are gluten-free doesn't guarantee that they are low in calories, fat, sugar or salt.
• Decreasing the amount of carbohydrates in your diet may encourage you to eat more fruit and vegetables.	• Because gluten provides flavour to the foods in which it is naturally found, removing the gluten also removes the signature taste that many people love in, for instance, bread products.
	• It's expensive – gluten-free foods can cost two to three times more.

Personality: You're highly analytical and love detail. Ensuring zero gluten sneaks onto your plate is your kind of challenge.

Body shape: Well cushioned – having a cushiony layer all over your frame is a sign of water retention, which could be linked to intolerance to gluten.

Any health concerns?

While experts agree that a gluten-free diet is important for sufferers of coeliac disease, there is no real evidence that it will help people who aren't gluten intolerant to lose weight – or, indeed, if it's even healthy for non-coeliacs to cut gluten out of their diet.

The view of most dieticians is that there's nothing magical about eliminating gluten that results in weight loss, as replacing cakes, bread and pasta with fruit and veg is bound to help you shed pounds because you're generally going to be consuming fewer calories.

There is also the danger that a gluten-free diet could be unhealthier than your normal diet because gluten-free versions of favourite food products often have a higher sugar and fat content to make them taste better. A *Sunday Times* newspaper survey of gluten-free products from four big supermarkets found that most were considerably higher in fat than the equivalent standard product. A bowl of gluten-free granola from one shop contained more fat than a Mars bar (Milky Way).

Wholegrain wheat, rye and barley are also full of fibre and important nutrients, so gluten-free dieters who rely on replacement products can end up eating a lot of food that is "stripped" of important goodness such as fibre and iron. Because it's such a restrictive diet, you should also consult your doctor before going gluten free.

Want to know more?

Read: *Gluten-Free Girl Every Day* by Shauna Ahern (John Wiley & Sons, 2013).

The Grapefruit Diet

One of the first diet fads, based on the belief that eating the popular breakfast fruit as often as possible will burn off fat.

The weight-loss promise:
Lose 10 lb (4.5 kg) in just 10–12 days.

The Grapefruit Diet has existed since at least the 1930s, when it was so popular among wannabe movie starlets that it was known as the Hollywood Diet. Its fame continued to grow as the masses followed in the footsteps of their idols and started trying to lose weight on this particular diet craze.

The plan resurfaced much later in the 1970s, when the details were faxed between followers, along with the claim that grapefruit was a miracle weight-loss cure that had the ability to melt away fat. It continued to be popular into the 1980s, when it became known as the "10-day 10-pounds-off Diet". As a result, for many women losing weight in the seventies and eighties was synonymous with gorging on grapefruits!

Interest was reignited in the potential of grapefruits to aid weight loss this century thanks to a 2003 study at the Scripps Clinic in California. The research aim was to measure the effectiveness of grapefruit in treating insulin resistance and lowering weight in overweight patients who were not otherwise trying to diet. The successful study received considerable publicity and revived interest in incorporating grapefruit into weight-reduction diets. The study used grapefruit in capsule form as well as fresh grapefruit – a fact that prompted the development of several over-the-counter "miracle" diet pills containing grapefruit extract.

The plan

The first versions of the Grapefruit Diet lasted for seven days and were extremely low-calorie diets, with the dieter consuming little except black coffee and half a grapefruit at each meal, plus small amounts of salad and lean meat.

By the 1970s, the Grapefruit Diet had become high protein and involved eating half a grapefruit before each meal and consuming just 800 calories a day for 10–12 days, followed by two days off. This regime was then repeated until the desired weight was reached. In effect, it's a very low-calorie and low-carb diet, which involves giving up sugar, sweet fruits and vegetables, bread, coffee, grains and cereals. It encourages the consumption of meat, eggs and other foods that are rich in fat and protein, and you can prepare food using any cooking method you like, including frying.

Exercise isn't generally recommended because you're consuming so few calories.

How it works

The diet is based on the idea that, when consumed before meals, a special enzyme in grapefruit turns the body into a fat-burning machine. It's further suggested that grapefruit helps burn even more body fat when eaten with foods high in fat and protein.

The researchers behind the more recent Scripps Clinic study certainly believe grapefruit contains unique plant compounds that reduce insulin levels, which, in turn, promotes weight loss. But the reason for this effect is as yet unclear. High levels of insulin can indicate that sugar isn't efficiently being utilized for energy, with the result that it's more likely to be stored as fat. But high levels of insulin can also make

DAILY MENU EXAMPLE	
Breakfast	½ grapefruit, 2 slices of bacon, 2 boiled eggs, black coffee (no sugar) or unsweetened tea
Lunch	½ grapefruit, small salad with low-calorie dressing, lean chicken, black coffee or unsweetened tea
Dinner	½ grapefruit, salad with low-calorie dressing, 8 oz (225 g) lean chicken, lean beef or fish, black coffee or unsweetened tea

people feel hungry so that they eat more. Finally, high levels of insulin prevent the body from breaking down fat. What exactly it is in grapefruit that has this insulin-lowering effect has yet to be isolated.

Who is it best for?

Lifestyle: You don't have too many responsibilities, such as kids or a demanding job, so feeling a little low in energy won't disrupt your day.

Personality: You're good at following rules and don't give up easily, but want fast results.

Body shape: Plus size – this diet doesn't include any toning exercises, so it isn't going to help you tone up or focus on specific problem areas; you will lose weight all over.

PROS	CONS
• Eating half a grapefruit before meals could help ensure you eat fewer calories during the rest of the meal.	• Unfortunately, the results aren't likely to last. As with all crash diets, the weight you lose is mostly fluid, and because you don't change your long-term eating habits, there's a good chance you'll regain it.
• Grapefruit is a very low-calorie fruit (66–84 calories per serving), plus it's loaded with vitamin C and fibre.	
• Because the daily calories are very low – averaging 800–1,000 in most versions – most people will lose weight on this plan.	• This diet doesn't allow sufficient calories to supply the daily energy needs of even a moderately active adult and is nutritionally insufficient.
	• The variety of food you're allowed to eat is very limited, meaning it's easy to get bored and crave more interesting foods.

Any health concerns?

Most experts say that all versions of this diet remain far too low in calories for sustainable, healthy weight loss, and the diet plan lacks essential nutrients and fibre. Even the researcher who designed and conducted the Scripps Clinic trial has specifically warned people against very low-calorie Grapefruit Diets, saying that they are unhealthy.

And despite the Scripps Clinic study, the jury is still out as to whether grapefruit has any special fat-burning properties, as it was only a small-scale study, and most nutrition experts feel one study is not enough to pin magical weight-loss powers on a fruit. Any initial weight loss following this plan is due to draining the body's carbohydrate stores, fluid loss and the inevitable reduction in your overall calorie intake, rather than the purported "fat-burning" ability of grapefruit. The diet does not allow you to establish longer-term healthy-eating changes so the weight may easily be regained.

A Grapefruit Diet can also be harmful if you're taking any of the medications, including the cholesterol-lowering drugs statins, that interact with grapefruit, according to recent studies. Always consult your doctor before starting any low-calorie diet, especially if you're on medication.

Want to know more?

Read: *The Grapefruit Solution: Lower Your Cholesterol, Lose Weight and Achieve Optimal Health with Nature's Wonder Fruit* by Daryl Thompson and M. Joseph Ahrens (LINX Corp, 2004).

The Hay Diet

Stop eating proteins and carbs at the same time and you'll stay slim for ever.

The weight-loss promise:
You'll improve the body's natural ability to digest foods, which will help you lose weight and ease health conditions such as IBS.

The Hay Diet was first created by New York doctor William Howard Hay in the 1920s. Dr Hay developed his diet as an attempt to improve his health after he was diagnosed with a kidney-related condition called Bright's disease, high blood pressure and a dilated heart. He decided to treat his symptoms by creating a healthy eating plan and found he experienced a reduction of symptoms as well as incidentally losing weight.

Hay spent the following decade studying food in a bid to reduce the acidic "end product" of digestion, which he believed to be the cause of many health problems. He found that fruits and vegetables produce an alkaline end product when broken down in the stomach, while processed foods produce acid. He went on to invent the concept of food-combining, believing that eating certain foods together would cause even alkaline foods to trigger an undesirable acidic digestion. The resulting Hay Diet has seen a resurgence in popularity in recent years, with several high-profile celebrities said to be fans.

The plan

The major rule is that no meal should contain both protein and carbohydrates. Food is also grouped into two further categories, alkaline and acidic, with acid foods not to be combined with alkaline ones. It should be noted that Hay's use of these terms does not completely conform to the more scientific pH of the foods: the acidic foods he selects tend to be protein-rich, such as meat, fish, dairy, while Hay's alkaline foods are carbohydrate-rich, such as rice, grains and potatoes.

Dr Hay suggested that the ideal meal should consist of alkaline-forming foods and acid-forming foods at the ratio of about four to one in favour of alkaline. Of your three meals a day, one should contain only alkaline foods; meal two, protein foods with salads, vegetables and fruit; and the third, starchy carbs with salads, vegetables and sweet fruit. There should be an interval of four to four and a half hours between each meal.

Vegetables, salads and fruits comprise the major part of the diet. Proteins, starches and fats need to be eaten in small quantities, and you should also cut down on the amount of meat you eat. All refined and processed foods should be eliminated from the diet, and only whole grains and unprocessed starches eaten.

Exercise

Dr Hay believed that exercise did not provide the answer to weight loss or healthy digestion. Speaking from an earlier age, Hay pointed out that farmers who were physically active were diagnosed with some of the same conditions that less sedentary people were!

How it works

At the root of the Hay Diet is the idea, so far unsupported by science, that certain diseases develop because the chemicals in a person's body are poorly balanced as a direct result of

DAILY MENU EXAMPLE	
Breakfast	Orange juice and milk
Lunch	Tomato soup, a baked onion, a tomato-and-cucumber salad with mayonnaise dressing; apricots for dessert
Dinner	Grilled (broiled) fish or steak, steamed chicory, steamed carrots, and a salad of shredded cabbage, onions and radishes, with mayonnaise dressing, followed by lemon sorbet

acidic substances created during digestion. Hay felt that this created a deficit of necessary alkaline substances, leading to health problems such as indigestion and obesity. To reduce these so-called "acid end products" Hay argued that a dieter should avoid overeating meat and refined carbohydrates and stop combining incompatible foods.

For example, he claimed: "Any carbohydrate foods require alkaline conditions for their complete digestion, so must not be combined with acids of any kind, such as sour fruits, because the acid will neutralize the alkaline. Neither should these be combined with a protein of a concentrated sort as these protein foods will excite too much hydrochloric acid during their stomach digestion."

Hay felt that if you followed the food-combining rules and avoided eating protein and carbohydrates at the same time, your stomach would digest food more easily, thus preventing weight gain and other health problems.

PROS	CONS
• You generally don't have to stop eating the foods you enjoy – just change when and how you eat them.	• It's almost impossible to completely avoid mixing carbs and protein, as most foods contain a little of both.
• You don't need to starve yourself in order to get results. Fans have said they eat more on the Hay Diet and still lose weight.	• Hay's theory of digestion isn't backed by the scientific community.
• It is likely that you'll increase your intake of healthy whole grains, fruit and vegetables.	• You may experience carbohydrate cravings after protein meals, which will make this diet difficult to stick to.
	• Family meals and eating out are extremely tricky on this diet.

Who is it best for?

Lifestyle: You're most at home in the kitchen and are happy to spend a lot of time here, thinking about creating meals that combine only certain foods.

Personality: You're a planner who will happily ponder the contents of each meal. You crave order and are happiest when everything is in its correct place.

Body shape: Curvy – the diet was created in the 1920s to narrow women down into the flapper silhouette: slim-hipped and small-chested.

Any health concerns?

The theory that carbohydrate- and protein-rich foods should be eaten separately for better digestion is considered unfounded by most mainstream nutritionists. They point out that Hay conveniently ignores the fact that carbohydrate-rich foods all contain significant amounts of protein. Eating protein separately from carbohydrates also tends to cause the body to burn the protein as an energy source, rather than to build muscle.

Nor is there any scientific evidence to suggest that the body can't digest different food groups at the same time. The body has different digestive enzymes, such as amylase in the mouth for digesting carbohydrates, and peptins in the stomach for digesting proteins. Short of a medical condition, one enzyme shouldn't interfere with the other. As a result, there's also no evidence to suggest that consuming carbohydrates separately from proteins will have any influence on weight loss. That said, anyone trying to separate food groups at mealtimes, as Hay suggests, is likely to consume fewer overall calories, not least because it's pretty hard to follow.

Want to know more?

Read: *Food Combining for Health: The Original Hay Diet* by Doris Grant and Jean Joice (Thorsons, 2004).

The Hypno Diet

With the help of hypnotherapy, you can literally think yourself thin.

The weight-loss promise:
By reprogramming your mind to enjoy healthy food and make healthier choices, you'll reach and maintain your target weight without hunger, guilt or stress.

The use of hypnosis for therapeutic purposes dates back as far as the ancient Egyptians. But it was in the twentieth century that the two worlds of psychology and hypnosis crossed paths to form hypnotherapy – a treatment used to tap into a patient's subconscious in order to create a change in thoughts and associated behaviour. It didn't take long for advocates to suggest that hypnotherapy might be a way to alter a person's unhealthy eating habits.

In 1999, the British Medical Journal published a clinical review of current medical research, which concluded: "A systematic review has found that hypnosis enhances the effects of cognitive behavioural therapy for conditions such as phobia, obesity and anxiety."

Hypno-dieting received perhaps its biggest PR boost in the UK in 2009 when singer Lily Allen told journalists how it had helped her shrink from a UK size 14 to a size 8 (US size 10 to 4). She revealed that the secret to her weight loss was that she'd had her brain reprogrammed, by Susan Hepburn, a hypnotherapist from London's Harley Street, to encourage her to exercise more and remove the desire to eat fattening foods.

The plan

Not technically a diet, hypno-dieting is a way of encouraging your mind to make healthier food choices. The first thing the hypnotherapist is likely to ask you to do is to keep a food diary in which you write down everything you eat. You will then use it to identify the reasons you eat when you're not hungry: is it boredom, stress or sadness that makes you turn to the biscuit tin (cookie jar)? You will also talk through your body image.

Once you've pinpointed all the emotional triggers that make you turn to food, the next stage is to try to improve your eating habits. The aim is to replace fattening behaviours with healthier ones that allow you to lose weight. Through the power of suggestion, the hypnotherapist will help you to learn to eat only when your body needs to eat; desire foods that are healthy; choose to stop when your body is full; eat slowly and mindfully; and to re-introduce exercise into your life. During the sessions, you will be asked to visualize yourself slim and to focus on this goal. A course of sessions is usually required.

Exercise

In the same way that the hypno diet can help reprogramme your mind to make better food choices, it can also help encourage you to make healthier lifestyle decisions overall, for example, creating more positive associations with exercise, therefore boosting your motivation to work out.

How it works

The "hypno" part is claimed to work because, in a state of hypnosis, you're focused and calm and your subconscious is more receptive to ideas and suggestions. The therapy is then based on the principal of "behavioural change through positive reinforcement". Rather than telling yourself what you're "not" allowed to eat, you teach your subconscious that what you really want is healthy food and exercise.

Susan Hepburn explains: "When you're in this state of deep relaxation (hypnosis), it's possible to bypass the conscious mind and reach the more 'suggestible' subconscious. This part of your mind holds the deep-rooted habits, beliefs and impulses that undermine your best intentions.

"I liken it to deleting unwanted files from a computer. First you remove from your subconscious mind the emotional associations that cause you to eat when you're not hungry.

PROS	CONS
• It supposedly bypasses willpower. • You shouldn't feel hungry on this diet. • You shouldn't experience cravings, as hypno-dieting attempts to break the hold unhealthy foods have over you, so you'll no longer yearn for them. • Unlike other diet plans that last for a set amount of time and then leave you to go back to your old eating habits, hypno-dieting should change your eating habits for life.	• Although it sounds very easy, hypnosis alone won't help you lose weight unless you're prepared to make the lifestyle changes as well. • There's no suggested eating plan in this diet, so it won't be for you if you would like more guidance. • Although hypnosis is an ancient concept, hypno-dieting has only been around for a short time and not much is known about its long-term success rate.

Next you reprogramme your mind with healthy and positive attitudes to food and exercise."

Hypno-dieting also encourages you to eat mindfully – to really savour food, so that you enjoy and get the most out of eating, becoming more aware of what you put in your body and making healthier choices as a result.

Who is it best for?

Lifestyle: Busy. You always have a million and one things going on, so there's no time to plan what you are eating, and you tend to eat unhealthy food mindlessly.

Personality: You have an addictive personality and little willpower, and have developed unhealthy eating habits that you feel unable to tackle – whether it be turning to chocolate for comfort or indulging in takeaways after a stressful day at work. You may also be a yo-yo dieter with a history of failing to stick to diets.

Body shape: You're carrying too much weight all over and desperately want to shed at least 2 stone (28 lb/13 kg).

Any health concerns?

Hypno-dieting is still considered a fairly controversial therapy, as many health professionals dispute its effectiveness. Hypnotherapy is, however, endorsed by the NHS in the UK as one of the complementary and alternative medicines that can be considered for obesity.

If you have any pre-existing health conditions or mental health problems, talk to your GP first, and make sure your hypnotherapist is trained in working with your particular condition. Results tend to depend on the hypnotherapist and your relationship with them. It's also critical they provide sound nutritional advice to you in a suggestible state. In other words, it's a good idea to ask about their healthy-eating views beforehand. It's also vital to check any therapist credentials thoroughly – at the very least making sure that they belong to an appropriate professional body – because there are some non-professionals with little training who also offer this service. A therapist recommended by a trusted friend is also worth seeking out.

Want to know more?

Read: *Hypnodiet: Lose Weight, Feel Fabulous – the Stress-Free Way* by Susan Hepburn (Piatkus, 2010).

The Macrobiotic Diet

Eating nothing but raw food will lead to health gains and weight loss.

The weight-loss promise:
You'll enjoy better health. There are no weight-loss promises attached to this diet, however the strict food rules mean followers are likely to lose excess weight.

The word "macrobiotic" has Greek roots and means "long life" but it was Japanese philosopher and teacher George Ohsawa who, in the 1930s, created the basis of what we now know as macrobiotic eating. He believed simplicity in diet was the key to good health and that avoiding certain foods could even cure cancer and other serious illnesses. In practice, this meant lots of raw and organic fruit and veg. Ohsawa was an early advocate of organic agriculture, regional food production, seasonal eating and reducing or eliminating animal foods from the diet. His recommended diet involves 10 stages that grow progressively more restrictive.

Macrobiotics was introduced to the UK in 1966, when a young American named Craig Sams moved to London to open the UK's first macrobiotic restaurant, Seed. But it was in the 1990s that the Macrobiotic Diet truly hit the mainstream when A-list celebrities, including Gwyneth Paltrow, Julia Roberts and Madonna, admitted they had tried it out.

The plan

You stick to a low-fat, high-fibre diet consisting of around 50 per cent whole grains, such as brown rice and buckwheat pasta, 20–30 per cent vegetables, 5–10 per cent beans and sea vegetables, 5–10 per cent miso soup and 5 per cent condiments and supplementary foods, including drinks, fish and desserts. Other elements may include occasional helpings of nuts, seeds, pickles and non-stimulating and non-aromatic teas. All food should be locally and organically grown.

The plan also involves avoiding the "toxins" that come from eating dairy products, meats, eggs, coffee, sugar, stimulants and aromatic herbs, and processed or refined foods. Some vegetables including potatoes, tomatoes, aubergine (eggplant), peppers, asparagus, spinach and avocados are also discouraged and should only be used sparingly.

Food should be mainly raw or lightly steamed. Pots, pans and utensils should only be made from wood, glass, ceramic or stainless steel, and microwaves and vitamin and mineral supplements are banned. Other rules include eating only when hungry, chewing food thoroughly, eating in a relaxed manner – and always sitting with a good posture.

Exercise

Gentle yoga is recommended, as are daily walking and stretching exercises.

How it works

Macrobiotics is based on a belief that food has an invisible energy (yin and yang) that cannot be measured scientifically and which affects how healthy it is. Although all foods have both yin and yang qualities, some foods are seen as extremely yin, while others are extremely yang. According to macrobiotics, an imbalance of foods that are too yin or too yang can lead to illness.

Whole grains such as brown rice are seen as very balanced foods, so the more of them you eat, the easier it is to balance yin and yang in your diet as a whole. Another important rule is to eat food local to you. This is based on the idea that good health depends on our evolutionary ability to adapt to fit our local environment, and if we eat foods from a climate that is very different from ours, our bodies struggle to digest them. Evidence for this is based on the fact that most cultures that have moved away from their traditional diet have historically experienced a corresponding rise in chronic illness.

Who is it best for?

Lifestyle: You live in the country and grow your own fruit and veg, or have access to local organic produce. You only work part-time or not at all, and have lots of time to prepare food.

Personality: You have a strong spiritual side, possibly with an interest in Eastern mysticism. You're a firm believer in

DAILY MENU EXAMPLE	
Breakfast	Vegetable and miso soup, brown rice with kombu (kelp) and shiitake mushrooms, green tea
Lunch	Udon noodles with steamed Brussel sprouts and salad, green tea
Dinner	Baked cod with ginger, green beans, watercress and blueberries, green tea

PROS	CONS
• Due to the emphasis on vegetables, fruits and whole grains, the Macrobiotic Diet contains a large amount of dietary fibre and is rich in many important vitamins and minerals.	• Banning meat and dairy products makes for a very limited vegan diet.
• This diet restricts the intake of saturated fat, cholesterol, sugar, alcohol, and processed foods, all of which are known to negatively impact health.	• The limit to locally grown foods will severely narrow down your food options.
	• The restrictions placed on cooking methods also limit your options when looking for recipes to fit the plan.
• With so many fibre-packed whole grains and veggies, you won't feel hungry.	• It's not just a diet – macrobiotics is a (very strict) way of life!

alternative medicine and are looking for a full health makeover, not just to drop a few pounds.

Body shape: Pear – it's harder to shift excess weight from your thighs and hips than from your middle. This diet is low in fat and high in healthy carbs, which may help to kick-start a sluggish metabolism.

Any health concerns?

Although following a Macrobiotic Diet at its most basic, near-vegan level can be good for you, if you work through all of Ohsawa's 10 different stages, cutting more and more foods out as you go, you could be doing yourself more harm than good. For example, avoiding meat and dairy could lead you to become low in vitamin B12, vitamin D, calcium, zinc and iron. Because of these potential deficiencies (supplements are also banned), this type of diet is definitely not suitable for children or for pregnant or breastfeeding women.

Although macrobiotics devotees present the lifestyle as a means of combating cancer, there is no robust scientific research to back this up, and both the American Cancer Society and Cancer Research UK actually recommend against cancer patients following the diet. This is because people suffering with cancer often have increased nutritional and calorie requirements so such a strict diet is not a sensible idea.

Needless to add, the idea of yin and yang in food is also disputed by scientists. Ultimately, and perhaps most importantly, it's such an extreme and strict diet, most people will struggle to follow it for more than a very short time.

Want to know more?

Read: *Modern Day Macrobiotics: Transform Your Diet and Feed Your Mind, Body and Spirit* by Simon Brown (Carroll & Brown, 2005).

The Mediterranean Diet

Eat Med-style with lots of olive oil, fish and veggies to enjoy a slimmer figure and longer life.

The weight-loss promise:
Following a Mediterranean Diet plan with controlled portions could result in slow and lasting weight loss of 1–2 lb (450–900 g) a week.

The health benefits of the Mediterranean Diet – the traditional diet of countries such as Italy, Spain, Southern France and Greece – were first publicized in 1945 by an American doctor called Ancel Keys. He had been living in Italy and observed the high concentration of centenarians and low rates of obesity. He put this squarely down to the fact that the Mediterranean Diet offered a range of health-protecting benefits.

Today, this traditional diet, rich in olive oil, fish and vegetables, is considered by many to be the healthiest diet in the world. Numerous studies have found it can lower your risk of heart disease and stroke, diabetes and certain cancers, plus it may help combat depression and ward off dementia. And, provided you exercise in moderation, it can also be an excellent weight-loss plan.

The plan

Rather than a strict "diet", this is more a change of lifestyle that leans towards making healthier food choices for ever, rather than quick fixes.

Mediterranean Diets are typically high in legumes (such as beans and peas), unrefined cereals, fish, olive oil, fruits and vegetables; they have a high monounsaturated fat to saturated fat ratio; include a moderate alcohol (mainly red wine) and dairy product intake; and are low in meat and meat products. Additionally, the Mediterranean lifestyle includes leisurely dining and regular physical activity. Most foods included in the Mediterranean Diet are fresh and seasonal, rather than highly processed. Preparation methods tend to be simple – foods are rarely deep-fried.

Exercise

Regular physical activity has always been a traditional part of rural life in the Med, but nothing too fast and furious due to the intense summer heat. Thirty minutes of brisk walking a day is recommended.

How it works

The benefits of the Mediterranean Diet are based on what, from the point of view of mainstream nutrition, is considered a paradox: although traditional Mediterranean inhabitants tend to consume relatively high amounts of fat, they have far lower rates of cardiovascular disease and obesity than in countries like the UK and USA. Nutritionists believe that it must be the types of fat consumed that account for this paradox. In the UK and USA, people tend to consume a larger amount of trans and saturated fats, while in the Mediterranean countries they tend to eat mainly monounsaturated and polyunsaturated fats – from olive oil and fish – which lower cholesterol.

The Mediterranean Diet also includes plenty of foods that are rich in lean protein and fibre (such as beans and pulses), which are filling and therefore more satisfying. Red wine, which is traditionally served in moderation at mealtimes, is also considered a health plus, because it contains flavonoids with powerful disease-fighting antioxidant properties.

The Mediterranean way of life also encourages taking time over meals, which has also been shown to reduce the likelihood of obesity. A study presented at the North American Association for the Study of Obesity showed that overweight men and women took in fewer calories when they slowed their normal eating pace.

Who is it best for?

Lifestyle: Busy and sociable, with a diary full of dinner dates and evening drinks.

DAILY MENU EXAMPLE	
Breakfast	Greek yogurt with berries and a handful of nuts, fruit juice
Morning snack	Apple
Lunch	Lentil or bean soup served with tomato and feta salad and olive oil
Afternoon snack	Nuts and olives
Dinner	Grilled (broiled) chicken or fish served with roasted Mediterranean vegetables such as courgettes (zucchini), peppers and aubergine (eggplant), drizzled with lemon juice and olive oil. Glass of red wine

PROS	CONS
• You don't have to cut out any of the major food groups.	• The Mediterranean diet can be high in salt – foods such as olives, salt-cured cheeses, hams, anchovies, capers and salted nuts.
• It's a healthy food plan for life, not just for weight loss.	
• You can enjoy a glass of wine with dinner.	• You'll need to be careful about portion sizes, especially for higher-calorie foods such as nuts and olive oil.
• This diet is simple, so even reluctant cooks will be able to create dishes that fit the diet plan.	
• The wide variety of Mediterranean foods available makes it easy to continue following the diet long term.	• You won't get to eat much red meat.

Personality: You're a straight talker who has no time for gimmicks. You also have no patience for feeling deprived and so need a diet that doesn't ban foods or severely restrict calories. You may also be drawn to the relaxed and social Mediterranean way of life generally.

Body shape: Narrow-framed, with similar breadth shoulders and hips, but a tendency to gain weight around the middle, which can lead to a higher risk of heart disease. The Mediterranean Diet incorporates healthy fats that can help decrease your risk of cardiovascular problems.

Any health concerns?

Although this is considered to be one of the healthiest diets in the world by many health experts, it is advised that you keep a watchful eye on serving sizes of fats and oils. Even though unsaturated fats are healthy, don't go overboard, or you'll struggle to consume fewer calories than you burn. The key, as with the recommendations on red wine, is moderation. Because there isn't specific guidance on portion sizes and calorie intakes, you will need to work this out yourself to avoid over-consumption.

Another minor point of contention may be that this diet plan advises against eating many potatoes, when there is no scientifically proven reason to do so. One medium-sized baked potato with skin has just 200 calories and is virtually fat-free. Potatoes are a good source of fibre, iron, phosphorus, vitamin B6 and niacin, and a fair source of vitamin C, and if cooked in a healthy way, are pretty good for you.

Want to know more?

Read: *The Greek Doctor's Diet* by Dr Fedon Alexander Lindberg (Rodale International Ltd, 2006).

The Nordic Diet

Enjoy a smorgasbord of Scandinavian goodies and fit back into your jeans in no time.

The weight-loss promise:
A balanced, high-protein diet that's full of fresh food, simply prepared, which will help keep you slim for the long term.

In recent years, a lot of interest has been paid to the traditional foods from the group of Nordic countries that includes Sweden, Norway, Denmark and Finland. Some experts now think this north European diet could be just as good for slimming and overall health as the more famous southern European "Mediterranean Diet".

The benefits are thought to be down to the natural goodness of local Nordic fare – foods such as low-fat dairy, fish, red meat, berries and rye bread. Add to this a culinary culture that favours smaller portions and an active lifestyle and it becomes clear why people from these countries have both low levels of obesity and long life expectancies.

The plan

Sticking to a Nordic Diet means eating plenty of the following traditional foods.

Berries: Numerous studies have found that berries, a Nordic staple, are packed with vitamins and antioxidants that help prevent disease and premature ageing.

Rapeseed oil: Also called canola oil, this is used as a cooking fat, replacing alternatives like olive oil. Rapeseed is very rich in omega-3 oils as well as vitamin E.

Leafy green veg: Cabbage, Brussels sprouts and kale are key, and they are all packed with B vitamins and disease-fighting antioxidants.

Oily fish: Salmon, mackerel and herring are good examples of the fish that are prominent in the Nordic Diet. They contain omega-3s, which are good for the heart as well as possibly preventing some forms of cancer.

Lean red meat, especially game: Full of iron and able to provide long-lasting energy, gamey meats like duck or venison tend to be lower in fat because the animals lived wild and had the chance to run around.

Rye bread: Made with the whole grain, rye bread is packed with fibre and won't cause the sharp rises in blood sugar associated with wheat-based breads that create food cravings.

On the Nordic Diet you're encouraged to eat little and often, opting for up to five or six smaller meals over three big ones. This falls in line with a popular theory among nutritionists that grazing keeps your metabolism ticking over, meaning your body burns off calories more effectively so that less are stored as fat. Eating at the table as a family and taking your time over food is also recommended.

Exercise

Nordic dieters are recommended to do at least 30 minutes exercise every day. In Scandinavia this usually means enjoying the outdoor life and maintaining a connection with nature by walking, swimming or cycling. Indeed, cycling is often the preferred means of transportation in both cities and the countryside.

How it works

The Nordic Diet is high in protein diet but there is a particular focus on lean game meats and fish. The diet is also incredibly high in antioxidant-rich fruit and vegetables. According to Professor Astrup from the University of Copenhagen in Denmark: "There's increasing evidence that the fat in meat is not as unhealthy as we are led to believe. The protein content of low-fat dairy products, healthy fish and lean game is very beneficial if you want to feel full for fewer calories. To maintain a healthy body weight, these parts of the diet should not be excluded."

DAILY MENU EXAMPLE	
Breakfast	Smoked trout and granary toast
Lunch	Pickled herring salad with a sliced apple and boiled egg
Snack	Rye crispbread with tuna
Dinner	Venison sausages with mash, plus cooked cabbage. Bowl of mixed berries

PROS	CONS
• If you buy a good Nordic Diet book with lots of recipes, it will feel less like a diet and more like an exploration of a new cuisine.	• It can be time-consuming and expensive to source fresh Nordic ingredients. You also need to enjoy cooking.
• A recent study by Lund University in Sweden, published in 2013, found that the Nordic Diet could lower cholesterol.	• Some foods might not be readily available outside of Scandinavia.
• Eating little and often accords with the health advice from many prominent nutritionists.	• You may find eating smaller, more regular meals tricky to fit in to your day.

In a small study of 250 men and women, Professor Astrup found that protein's ability to make us feel fuller for longer and speed up the metabolism meant that a high-protein diet was more effective in helping slimmers keep the weight off than the popular GI diet.

Who is it best for?

Lifestyle: You have plenty of time to shop, cook and eat out. You have a flexible daily schedule and no issues with eating early or late, so that five mealtimes a day is not a problem.

Personality: You're sociable, experimental and enjoy meals as an important part of family and social life. You want to lose weight but still want to enjoy what you eat. You're active, interested in nature and care about the provenance of food.

Body shape: You have a stone (14 lb/6 kg) or so to lose, or you carry weight around your middle, putting you at a higher risk of heart disease – something that this diet claims to address.

Any health concerns?

Because this diet is completely free of processed foods and, instead, focuses on natural produce such as nuts, berries and grains, it's a pretty healthy plan that could help reduce your risk of obesity and certain diseases. However, it does recommend relatively high levels of red meat, which has been associated with an increased risk of heart disease and bowel cancer, so going overboard with game could offset the benefits that you'll get from the other dietary components of the Nordic Diet.

Want to know more?

Read: *The Nordic Diet* by Trina Hahnemann (Quadrille, 2010).

The Paleo Diet

Stay slim, like a caveman, on the meat-heavy diet of our prehistoric ancestors.

The weight-loss promise:
Lose up to 75 lb (34 kg) in six months and enjoy optimal health on the diet we were designed to eat.

Gastroenterologist Walter L. Voegtlin was one of the first to suggest that following a diet similar to that eaten by our Palaeolithic ancestors would improve a person's health. In 1975, he self-published *The Stone Age Diet*, in which he argued that our ancestral diet was basically carnivorous – containing lots of fats and protein, with only small amounts of carbohydrates. Based on his own treatments of various digestive problems, including irritable bowel syndrome and indigestion, he claimed that by eating mainly meat and fish, along with fresh fruits and non-starchy vegetables, you could lose weight and prevent a range of illnesses. In the last 10 years, there has been a renewed interest in the so-called Paleo or "caveman" way of eating – with a raft of new diet books recommending this prehistoric eating plan as a way to keep slim.

The plan

In theory, you follow a hunter-gatherer diet consisting of similar wild plants and animals to those consumed during the Palaeolithic era – before the development of agriculture changed our diets.

In practice, this means eating organic foods that can be hunted and fished, such as fish, free-range meat, seafood and offal, as well as food that can be gathered, such as eggs, vegetables, fruit, seeds, nuts, herbs and spices. Food groups that, according to advocates of the diet, were rarely or never consumed by humans before the agricultural revolution are excluded from the diet. These are mainly grains, pulses, potatoes, dairy products, refined sugar and processed oil. In addition, any food product that includes chemicals you can't pronounce on its ingredient's list is off the menu.

Dieters must avoid salt and sugar. You can satisfy your sweet tooth with raw honey or coconut palm sugar, but only in limited quantities. Dieters must drink mainly water and no alcohol.

Exercise

The Paleo Diet encourages plenty of exercise, as it believes human bodies evolved to expect a certain level of daily physical activity. This means we should all aim for at least 60 minutes a day of moderate-intensity exercise.

How it works

The diet is based on the premise that humans have barely changed biologically since the Palaeolithic era, so the ideal diet for modern health and wellbeing is one that closely resembles what our ancestors ate.

The argument runs that many "modern" diet staples, such as dairy, beans, cereals, alcohol, sugar and vegetable oils, change the body's metabolism in a negative way and can be linked to certain diseases, including type 2 diabetes, cancer, asthma, heart disease, depression and obesity. Sticking to a Paleo-type diet reduces these so-called "modern diseases".

DAILY MENU EXAMPLE	
Breakfast	2 eggs with bacon
Lunch	Grilled chicken strips and asparagus
Dinner	Rotisserie chicken with sliced apple

Proponents of the Paleo Diet also say it switches your body from a mainly carb-burning machine to a fat-burning machine. This, they say, is ideal because your body's preferred source of energy is fats, as it's a much slower-burning fuel and more efficient. However, due to the abundance of carbohydrates that is eaten on a daily basis in the modern world, our body burns the quick-burning carbohydrates rather than fat. So, when we take in more carbohydrates than we need for energy, our body simply stores the excess as fat. The Paleo Diet changes this by removing a lot of the sugary carbohydrates from your diet. When this happens, your body can no longer get away with using carbs for energy and is forced to use fat stores instead – thus shifting excess weight.

Who is it best for?

Lifestyle: Active. You burn off a lot of energy as you perform all tasks with gusto, and you don't shy away from exercise or hard graft – you'd rather walk than drive. Also, to fit in the required amount of exercise, you will probably need to be doing some every day already.

PROS	CONS
• You can eat as much nutritious fruit and veg as you want.	• A true Palaeolithic diet is impossible to mimic because wild game isn't readily available, most other meats are domesticated and most modern plant food is cultivated rather than wild.
• This diet is very low in salt – good news for your heart.	
• The diet is high in energy-boosting iron.	
• The high intake of proteins and fats should keep you feeling full between meals.	• The high meat content of this diet makes it expensive to follow and impossible for vegetarians or vegans.
	• Cutting out all post-Palaeolithic foods means giving up staples such as milk, cheese, bread, pasta and potatoes.
	• The high red-meat content of this diet can give some people digestive problems.

Personality: You're a traditionalist, who is resistant to change. You're also a very happy carnivore, interested in good animal husbandry and food provenance generally.

Body shape: Android – broad shoulders with an undefined waist. Androids need adequate protein in their diet. Too much carbohydrate-rich foods like bread, cookies, pasta and sugar cause fat accumulation around the abdomen.

Any health concerns?

Although, in theory, this may seem like a sensible diet, particularly when removing sugar and salt, it cuts out several food groups, including dairy and grain, that provide essential nutrients, such as calcium, iron, vitamin D, magnesium, B vitamins and fibre. You could also end up eating a lot of artery-clogging saturated fat on the Paleo Diet, especially if you choose fatty cuts of meat. Plus, while the diet is high in fibre, thanks to the fruit and veg content, forbidden foods like whole-grain oats, beans and other grains are sources of soluble fibre, which have been found to help reduce high cholesterol levels and lower bowel cancer risk.

While there is some evidence to suggest we have problems digesting modern processed food, very few scientists would extend that group to include grains and plants like wheat that were first cultivated over 10,000 years ago. Overall, most dieticians agree that the Paleo Diet is neither sustainable nor healthy in the long term due to the lack of variety and the potential for nutrient deficiencies.

Want to know more?

Read: *The Paleo Diet: Lose Weight and Get Healthy by Eating the Foods You Were Designed to Eat* by Loren Cordain (John Wiley & Sons, 2010).

The Perricone Diet

Gorge on anti-inflammatory fish and berries for a slimmer body and more youthful skin.

The weight-loss promise:
"Lose weight and give yourself a natural facelift at the same time – all in just 72 hours."

Dr Perricone

Dr Nicholas Perricone is a dermatologist and nutritionist who has conducted a lot of research and written several books on the subjects of weight loss and maintaining a youthful appearance. He also has his own range of popular supplements and skin creams in the USA.

Dr Perricone first hit the headlines in the early noughties with his books *The Wrinkle Cure* and *The Perricone Prescription*, which claimed that a diet rich in salmon and berries could help you look younger within as little as three days – and drop excess pounds, too. He says his aim is to, "… lead to a change in our attitudes about how foods can affect health, beauty, longevity and wellbeing; critical changes needed to help save a society currently eating its way to poor health and obesity."

With a celebrity fan base said to include Cate Blanchett, Kim Cattrall, Uma Thurman and Julia Roberts, the Perricone brand is now big business.

The plan

Dr Perricone's anti-inflammatory diet consists of four main groups: high-quality protein, as found in fish, shellfish, poultry and tofu; low-glycaemic carbohydrates, including colourful fresh fruits and vegetables; whole grains such as oatmeal, legumes and lentils; and healthy fats, such as those found in cold-water fish (especially wild Alaskan salmon, halibut, sardines, herring, anchovies). In addition, you should eat nuts and seeds, cook in olive oil and drink 8–10 glasses of pure spring water per day, along with antioxidant-rich beverages such as green tea.

Perricone recommends five meals a day: breakfast, lunch, dinner and two snacks. He suggests you eat a lot from his list of superfoods and that you must always eat protein before you eat any carbohydrates. He advises cutting out foods that, he says, cause inflammation, such as alcohol, breads (especially French bread and croissants), flour, coffee, breakfast cereals (except porridge), duck, beef, fruit juice, fruits such as grapes, mangos, oranges, papaya, raisins, watermelon, many vegetables such as carrots, corn, peas and potatoes, plus pasta, rice and noodles, sugar and hard cheeses.

Exercise

Perricone recommends exercising for at least 20–30 minutes every day.

How it works

Dr Perricone's fish-based diet is all about banishing inflammation in the body. He says his research has led him to the conclusion that cellular inflammation may be the underlying cause of skin-related problems like spots and wrinkles and many serious diseases. This inflammation is not the redness that is visible to the naked eye but rather a microscopic irritation that takes place in the cells.

Perricone says that foods with a high glycaemic index cause inflammation throughout the body and that bad food choices are directly responsible for wrinkles, obesity and degenerative diseases. His particular bugbear is sugar, which he believes can be "toxic", contributing not only to weight gain but to the damage of internal organs and joints. Like many of his claims, scientific evidence to support this is currently thin.

His diet cuts out refined sugars and any carbs high on the glycaemic index but is rich in fish containing the omega-3 fatty acids that he believes have an anti-inflammatory effect

DAILY EATING PLAN

Wake up and immediately have a glass of water.

Breakfast	3–4 oz (85–115 g) smoked Nova Scotia salmon, porridge sprinkled with cinnamon, blueberries and chia seeds. Green tea or water
Snack	Cup cucumber slices and 2 slices Cheddar cheese
Lunch	4–6 oz (115–175 g) grilled turkey burger (no bun) with lettuce and tomato, plus white bean, watercress and asparagus salad
Afternoon snack	2 oz (55 g) sliced turkey or chicken breast, 4 hazelnuts, 4 celery sticks
Dinner	2–6 oz (55–175 g) grilled salmon, homemade artichoke and watercress soup, steamed spinach. Green tea or water

THE PERRICONE DIET

PROS	CONS
• Some other experts agree inflammation is a serious health problem and may contribute to diseases like arthritis and heart disease.	• Perricone frequently talks about his own research, but very little of it has ever been published or reviewed by other experts.
• This diet helps regulate blood sugars, which can curb your appetite.	• The plan is highly restrictive, cutting out many food staples, so you may have trouble sticking to it.
• This diet is rich in healthy antioxidants.	• This diet is very time-consuming; you will have to spend a lot of time preparing the meals and taking supplements.
• Perricone's plan promises to tackle two problems at once: weight and skin.	• Eating this much salmon is expensive.

and will therefore help improve skin problems, fight weight gain and reduce your risk of disease.

Who is it best for?

Lifestyle: You have a lot of "me" time to spend preparing meals for yourself rather than your family. You may also live near the sea or a very good fish market!

Personality: You're a bit of a hippy and like the idea of a "natural", pure diet. You're not a big carnivore by nature. Perhaps you were slim when younger but are a little concerned about the effects of getting older.

Body shape: You'd like to lose about a stone (14 lb/6 kg) and have problem skin.

Any health concerns?

Perricone's plan sounds healthy, but his underlying, and largely unsubstantiated, theory of inflammation produces some quirks. For instance, he claims that eating a Snickers bar would be preferable to a breakfast of orange juice, a bowl of cereal, a low-fat bran muffin with margarine and a cup of coffee – but there aren't many health experts who would agree with him! His diet also cuts out lots of nutritious foods such as dairy, certain fruit and veg and some cereals, which could lead to a lack of fibre and nutritional deficiencies.

Some doctors warn that such a protein-rich diet, apart from being expensive, could be unhealthy in the long term, and would be inadvisable for anyone with underlying kidney problems. Experts have also warned against eating too much fish, as it may be contaminated with high levels of mercury. On the plus side, Perricone's favourite, salmon, is one of the lowest risk fish for contamination. Current advice is that women of childbearing age should limit oily fish consumption to two portions a week because of concerns about the impact of low-level pollutants in the fish on a growing baby.

Perricone was once affiliated with Yale University School of Medicine but, along with most of the scientific establishment, the school authorities at Yale are now openly critical of both his books and his theories.

Want to know more?

Read: *The Perricone Weight-Loss Diet* by Dr Nicholas Perricone (Sphere, 2007).

The Personality Type Diet

Uncover your bad food habits to shed your "false weight" and stay slim long term.

> **The weight-loss promise:**
> Identify your personality traits and address bad habits and you'll both lose weight and keep it off in the long term.

The Personality Type Diet was created by Robert F. Kushner, a teacher of medicine at Northwestern University, Illinois, who had practical experience of treating obese patients. During clinics, he noticed the frustration that many dieters felt as they tried one diet after another without success and became certain that the common "one-size-fits-all" approach to losing weight was flawed. In Kushner's words: "As I paid more attention to my patient' symptoms of being overweight, I noticed definite patterns. One patient was a night eater, another used food to deal with stress, and yet another liked to exercise but couldn't fit it into her busy schedule." These different lifestyle patterns and how they could affect weight gain and diet success formed the basis of his book, *Dr. Kushner's Personality Type Diet*, first published in 2004.

The plan

Unlike most diets, which focus on food groups and meal plans, this approach focuses on the dieter. The first step is for dieters to understand how "scaling up" (unconscious eating, coping patterns) has impacted on their lives. This means looking back and asking if certain life events – such as the end of a relationship, quitting smoking, having kids or changing jobs – has triggered weight gain.

Once you've identified the common triggers of your weight gain, the next step is to answer a questionnaire about your habits and attitudes towards eating, which is designed to reveal your diet personality—you may be a night-time nibbler, a mindless muncher or a deprived sneaker. This helps you zero in on the lifestyle patterns that continually trip you up. Kushner then offers advice on how to overcome these traits and change your most troublesome behaviours and attitudes.

Week by week, dieters are encouraged to focus on making different areas of their life a better fit for their new approach to food in practical ways. First of all, he tackles the home environment – for example, by asking you to clear the cupboards of any problem foods, and to stock your fridge with healthy alternatives. Next, dieters are encouraged to "take control" of their daily activity by getting a pedometer and finding ways to bring more walking steps into their day. Finally, dieters must take control of their social life, and learn how to pick healthy meals when dining out.

There's no set meal plan or calorie counting. However, Kushner does advocate a largely vegetarian, low-fat diet, packed with certain "superfoods" including fruit, vegetables, grains, nuts, seeds, dried beans, lentils and soy products. Fish and poultry are on the menu but lean red meat should be eaten only in moderation.

Exercise

The plan also looks at your exercise personality to help find a way of working out to suit you.

How it works

Kushner believes that the answer to controlling weight once and for all doesn't lie in following a pre-printed diet plan or silly "food rules" but rather with having a better understanding of yourself and your particular lifestyle issues.

The diet centres on a condition called "scaling up syndrome", which Dr Kushner says must be treated before someone can lose weight for good. He blames this syndrome squarely on the pressures of modern life encouraging us to comfort eat as a coping strategy – made easier by the wide availability of cheap, convenient food. As a result, we pile on excess pounds, which he calls "false weight". "False weight is not weight resulting from genetics or metabolism or natural appetite or frame size or even low willpower," Kushner says. "It is weight resulting from an unconscious adaptation to the multifaceted pressures of modern society."

DAILY MENU EXAMPLE

The book does not offer a meal-by-meal diet. Instead, it offers tailored, easy-to-follow weight-loss tips for different personality types.

For the "Unguided Grazer"	Create a supporting structure; just eat – and enjoy; connect hunger and fullness cues; fill up on fibre and water
For the "Nighttime Nibbler"	Redistribute calories; calorie-proof your home; plan one nightly snack

PROS	CONS
• It's a bespoke diet just for you – you don't need to follow every rule in the book, just the ones that fit your "diet personality".	• The lack of a structured meal plan can make it difficult to follow this diet for those who like to have more guidance.
• It doesn't expect you to make lots of big changes quickly. It's divided up into small, manageable steps.	• Although it doesn't ban foods, don't be fooled into thinking this is an easy diet – behaviour change is hard work.
• It's not restrictive and includes a good balance of carbohydrates, proteins and fats.	• This diet doesn't offer a quick fix. Tackling deeper issues will take longer than simply reducing your calories to lose weight.
• It can help you identify the personality traits that may have derailed other diets in the past.	• Despite the tools in Kushner's book, emotional issues around food can be very difficult to diagnose and solve by yourself. You might find you also need expert advice in the form of a counsellor or psychologist.

The diet hinges on Kushner's theory that by becoming aware of the unhealthy food strategies we use to cope with life, we can form a healthier relationship with food and start to lose weight – and keep it off.

Who is it best for?

Lifestyle: All types – whether you are a busy office worker or retired with more time on your hands, this diet promises a plan designed to tackle your particular relationship with food.

Personality: Thoughtful – you're self-aware and like to work on improving yourself. You're independent and happy to handle the day-to-day business of eating more healthily yourself.

Body shape: All shapes and sizes. According to Kushner, storing fat in different regions of the body can be signs of different eating behaviours. This diet will target your specific problem and help you shed weight, regardless of body shape.

Any health concerns?

This plan makes few dietary stipulations, so there are no real nutritional problems to address. Research has shown that the best way to help someone achieve long-term weight loss is with bespoke advice and tailor-made plans, so this diet could be a useful place to start. Most experts agree that tackling underlying psychological attitudes to food is fundamental to long-term weight management. However, critics of this diet point out that, while Kushner is a well-respected nutrition expert, neither he nor his co-author – wife Nancy Kushner – are qualified psychologists. Most experts agree, though, that by and large the Kushners offer sound and sensible advice.

Want to know more?

Read: *Dr. Kushner's Personality Type Diet* by Dr Robert Kushner (iUniverse, 2008).

The Pritikin Program Diet

A very low-fat diet to reduce both your weight and your risk of heart disease.

The weight-loss promise:
A healthier, leaner, younger you – for years and years to come.

The Pritikin Program was originally founded in the 1970s by Nathan Pritikin, an American engineer who became interested in nutrition after he was diagnosed with advanced heart disease, aged just 41. The conventional medical wisdom for his diagnosis at the time was that nothing much could be done.

Unwilling to accept this advice, Pritikin studied cultures from around the world that had a very low incidence of heart disease and low cholesterol levels and used them to create his own low-fat diet and aerobic exercise regimen. After the approach apparently reversed Pritikin's own cardiac condition, the Pritikin Program was born.

The medical establishment was slow to credit Pritikin, who had no medical training, and some doctors criticized his diet as being unnecessarily severe. However, in 1976, the CBS television news programme *60 Minutes* followed three men, all with severe heart disease, as they attended the one-month programme at Pritikin's own diet centre. The show included extensive interviews with Pritikin and Dr David Lehr, a cardiologist from the Miami Heart Institute, who monitored the patients. All three improved dramatically.

As a consequence, Pritikin became a household name, and his theory that a healthy diet and exercise alone could beat obesity and prevent heart disease and diabetes became widely accepted, resulting in the bestselling book: *The Pritikin Program for Diet and Exercise* (1979).

Pritikin later developed leukaemia and eventually took his own life in 1985, aged 69, when his chemotherapy became too gruelling. However, following his death, the autopsy proved that he had in fact reversed his heart disease and had no plaque build-up in his arteries.

In recent years, Nathan's son Robert Pritikin has tweaked his father's diet concept, but the plan remains essentially low in fat and high in fibre.

The plan

Essentially, this a low-fat, low-salt, high-fibre plan. You eat mainly vegetables, fruit, whole grains and pulses, along with small amounts of low-fat dairy (or soy) products, fish and limited quantities of lean meat. Salt and refined grains, such as white pasta, white bread and white rice, are off the menu.

You don't have to count calories or measure portion sizes on this diet, but you do have to calculate the "average caloric density of your meal". The idea is to choose healthy foods that are not "calorie dense", meaning that they have relatively few calories per pound. For example, a pound of raw broccoli has just 130 calories, compared to a pound of chocolate-chip cookies, which has a whopping 2,140 calories.

To lose weight, most of us will need to keep the average calorific density of each meal below 880 calories per kilo. Since most vegetables fall below 440 calories per kilo, eating more of them will bring down the calorie average of each meal.

According to Pritikin's plan, by combining plenty of vegetables with the leanest portions of animal protein, it is possible to get the caloric density down to a level where you will lose weight. Dieters are also encouraged to eat smaller, more frequent meals instead of fewer larger ones.

Exercise

Exercise is a vital part of the plan, and Pritikin advises a three-pronged approach: 30–90 minutes a day of cardio exercise, such as swimming, cycling or walking, to burn calories; two to three sessions of strength training with weights each week, to burn fat and build more muscle; plus 10 minutes a day of stretching exercises, to keep your body flexible.

How it works

When the low-fat diet and aerobic exercise plan reversed his heart disease, it convinced Pritikin that "degenerative diseases are not diseases… they are environmental poisoning from the food we eat. Specifically toxic amounts of fat and cholesterol."

According to Pritikin, the typical Western diet is too high in cholesterol, fat, saturated and trans fats and salt. It's too low, meanwhile, in fibre and many important nutrients. A typical diet also includes an excess of nutrient-poor and calorie-dense foods such as sugar and other refined sweeteners, refined grains, refined fats and oils and alcohol. The Pritikin Eating Plan, on the other hand, is low in fat and salt and rich in natural unprocessed foods that are packed with vitamins, minerals, beneficial antioxidants and fibre, along with adequate amounts of protein and healthy fats.

Pritikin believed that we all have an evolutionary survival mechanism – dubbed our "fat instinct" – which makes us eat more than we need to, particularly fat; it also makes us store fat and take less exercise. All of this is to conserve our resources for leaner times – an ancient instinct that is both redundant and harmful in modern society. However, we can fool this instinct by limiting the fat we eat as much as possible and increasing the amount of fruit, veg and whole grains. These foods fill you up without the fat, giving you, he explained, "… the freedom to eat until you are full without limiting your portions or being hungry in order to lose weight."

Who is it best for?

Lifestyle: Those with a high-pressure lifestyle. The heart-healthy nature of this diet will help to counteract some of the strain put on your cardiovascular system from day to day. You may also have had a heart scare or suffer from stress.

DAILY MENU EXAMPLE	
Breakfast	Orange juice, wholegrain cereal, skimmed milk, plus a natural yogurt
Lunch	Lentil soup with wholegrain bread, broccoli salad and glass of skimmed milk
Snack	Raw carrots and celery
Dinner	Prawns (shrimp) and scallops stir-fry served with brown rice and steamed vegetables, plus 1 apple

PROS	CONS
• As well as helping weight loss, this diet brings a range of proven health benefits, including better heart health.	• It's a strict plan to follow.
	• The time commitment is high, especially if you stick to the daily exercise plan.
• It's vegetarian-friendly.	• The diet is incredibly low in fat and high in vegetables, which makes eating out rather difficult.
• You're encouraged to eat until you're full, so hunger should never be an issue.	• The very low quantity of fat can make meals a bit dry and not very tasty.

Personality: You're a mindless eater and tend to grab whatever's closest to hand without thinking about the effect it will have on your body. You also see food mainly as fuel, rather than something that should take time to prepare and savour. This plan will help you to start eating mindfully and change the way you view food.

Body shape: Apple – people who store fat around their middle are more at risk of cardiovascular disease, so have the most to gain from this diet plan.

Any health concerns?

The Pritikin Program is much higher in complex carbohydrates and much lower in fat than standard recommendations for healthy eating. The very limited amount of fats – including good or healthy fats such as those found in oily fish – could lead to deficiencies in essential fatty acids. Healthy fats such as omega-3s also help keep good cholesterol levels up and bad ones down. In addition, research now shows that some nutrients are better absorbed by the body when you're eating the recommended allowance of fat.

The low-meat and fat-free dairy requirements could also mean that you won't get enough vitamins D, E and B12 if you follow the diet to the letter. Restricting dairy products and therefore calcium in the long term can also increase the risk of the bone-thinning condition osteoporosis.

To summarize, there are probably alternative, more balanced plans that deliver the same health benefits without being quite so restrictive. The diet would be better for overall health and easier to maintain in the long term if it contained a slightly higher fat intake, provided this was mostly unsaturated fats.

Want to know more?

Visit: www.pritikin.com

The Raw Food Diet

If 75 per cent of your diet is raw fruit and veg, you will feel 100 per cent healthier and slimmer.

The weight-loss promise:
Eat a diet of mainly fruit and veg and you're likely to shed pounds at an unbelievable rate and enjoy fabulous health.

Dr Maximilian Bircher-Benner, the Swiss inventor of the breakfast favourite muesli, was one of the first people to recommend eating raw food to boost health and fight obesity back in the early 1900s. Believing raw apples had cured his own jaundice, Bircher-Benner conducted experiments into the effects of raw fruit and vegetables on human health. He concluded they could have a healing effect.

The Raw Food Diet gained mainstream popularity in 1984, when *Raw Energy: Eat Your Way to Radiant Health* by Leslie and Susannah Kenton was published. The book brought together years of research into raw foodism, citing examples such as the Hunza people from northern Pakistan whose sprouted seed-enriched diet is linked to their very long life expectancy. The Kentons' book recommends following a diet of 75 per cent raw food to stay slim, prevent degenerative diseases, slow the effects of ageing and boost energy levels.

In the past few decades, a host of celebrities have sung the praises of a Raw Food Diet, with Demi Moore, Uma Thurman, Susan Sarandon and Cher among those who have experimented with forms of the diet.

The plan

Raw foodists can be vegan, veggie or omnivores, so long as the food is raw and, ideally, organic. Any meat should be from free-range or grass-fed animals.

Your diet will consist of raw fruits, vegetables, nuts, seeds (including sprouted seeds) and eggs, raw fish (such as sashimi), raw meat (such as carpaccio) and non-pasteurized dairy products (such as raw milk, raw milk cheese and raw milk yogurt). Any nuts and seeds should be soaked overnight in water before eating to activate their enzymes.

You're allowed to eat food that has been "lightning cooked" at a temperature less than 40°C (104°F), but you will need to buy a special "dehydrator" machine for this. To prepare a varied Raw Food Diet, you will also need a blender, food processor and a juicer.

Coffee, alcohol and refined sugars, as well as tobacco, should be avoided, as should food that is processed or contains additives.

Exercise

Walking outdoors, yoga and meditation are recommended.

How it works

The fundamental principle behind raw foodism (or rawism) is that foods in their most natural state – uncooked and unprocessed – are best for the body because they contain natural enzymes, such as amylases, proteases and lipases, which are critical for good digestion. Heating or cooking food is thought to destroy these enzymes – and much of the food's nutritional content along with them. Raw fruits and vegetables are also high in antioxidants, and raw foodists believe this means that they can help to stifle signs of ageing and may have anti-cancer effects.

In addition, raw foods are believed to contain bacteria and other microorganisms that improve the immune system and digestion by populating the digestive tract with beneficial flora. Processed or cooked foods are thought to contain toxins,

DAILY MENU EXAMPLE	
Breakfast	Smoothie made with 1 banana, blueberries, strawberries, 1 tablespoon raw peanut butter, and raw cashew milk
Morning snack	Fruit salad made with a variety of seasonal produce, sprinkled with sliced almonds and raisins
Lunch	Homemade lentil houmous sandwich, with alfalfa sprouts, mixed greens, avocado, tomato and shredded carrots. The bread can be made from soaked buckwheat and sunflower seeds
Afternoon snack	1 pear and a homemade fruit and nut bar made with dates, raisins and raw almonds
Dinner	Courgette (zucchini) pasta with pesto – the "spaghetti" is shredded raw courgette, while ground cashews, garlic, lemon juice and basil leaves are used for the pesto. Side salad of rocket (arugula), spinach, celery, cucumbers, peppers, drizzled with olive oil and lemon
Dessert	Raw lime ice cream made with avocado, fresh lime juice, agave nectar and vanilla extract

PROS	CONS
• By placing an emphasis on plant foods, the diet is rich in nutrient-dense foods that are rich in fibre.	• You will miss out on the health benefits of some foods if you only eat them raw. Eggs, for instance, are a good source of biotin, a nutrient that is important for healthy hair, skin and bones. However, raw eggs contain a protein called avidin, which inactivates the biotin.
• The diet renounces processed foods, thus ditching most saturated fat, salt and sugar.	
• The strict food list means the total amount of calories you'll be able to eat on any given day will be low, so the pounds will drop off.	• Certain nutrient-rich foods cannot be eaten raw, such as beans and lentils.
	• The idea that cooking is "unnatural" is probably wrong. Humans cooked food long before the dawn of agriculture, suggesting that if cooking is unnatural, so is growing vegetables!
	• While eating uncooked foods is possible in summer, it's very hard in the winter.
	• Eating out is almost impossible.

which are not only fattening but can cause chronic disease, while heated fats such as fried oils are thought to be carcinogenic. Both these claims remain hotly disputed.

Who is it best for?

Lifestyle: You have plenty of time at home to prepare raw foods and don't work long hours. A home vegetable garden would also be useful.

Personality: You're a free-spirited child of nature, who likes the idea of a simple, organic way of living. Perhaps you have always wanted to live off the land and grow your own food. At the same time, you are very committed and willing to sacrifice favourite foods in a quest for better health.

Body shape: Pear – many pears have a problem with cellulite accumulating around the upper thighs and buttocks. Raw foodism advocates believe that a "toxin-free" diet that's high in antioxidants could improve cellulite.

Any health concerns?

While there is no doubt eating some foods raw can be healthy, there just isn't the scientific data to suggest that raw is always best. Or that cooking is as bad as claimed. For example, the idea that beneficial enzymes in plants are destroyed by cooking is undermined by the fact that the digestive process also destroys these same enzymes. Very few enzymes can survive hydrochloric acid in the stomach.

Some research has also shown that cooking certain vegetables, for example carrots, actually breaks down the cellular structure of the veg in a way that makes it easier for the body to absorb the nutrients they contain – especially if they are then served with a little olive oil or butter.

People following a Raw Food Diet, especially if it's vegetarian or vegan, need to make sure they're getting enough vitamin B12, calcium, iron and omega-3 fatty acids, nutrients that are most commonly found in animal products. It's also a good idea for people on this diet to increase their calcium intake, as the raw food staples like nuts and grains are high in sulphur-containing amino acids – which can increase bone calcium loss. If dairy-product consumption is reduced, then you may need to supplement with alternative sources such as green leafy vegetables, sesame seeds and almonds.

Eating raw meat, fish and dairy products also carries a higher-than-normal risk of food poisoning, because cooking or the pasteurization process kills most dangerous bacteria. This diet is therefore not safe for pregnant women, children or other at-risk groups.

Want to know more?

Read: *The Raw Food Detox Diet: The Five-step Plan for Vibrant Health and Maximum Weight Loss* by Natalia Rose (HarperCollins, 2006).

The Reverse Diet

Eat dinner for breakfast and your smallest meal in the evening to shed fat fast.

The weight-loss promise:
Eat dinner for breakfast and shed pounds, boost energy levels and enjoy better health. It's as simple as reversing your meals.

"Breakfast like a king, lunch like a prince, dine like a pauper" is age-old dietary advice but, since 2007, it has once again become a buzz phrase in weight-loss circles, thanks to the bestselling American diet book, *The Reverse Diet*.

The Reverse Diet is the creation of Tricia Cunningham, who teamed up with Heidi Skolnik, nutritionist for US Football team the New York Giants and the American School of Ballet, to produce the diet plan. Cunningham had battled with her weight for years and tried all sorts of diets to help her slim, but it was only when she tried simply reversing the order of her meals that she dropped half her body weight – losing more than 150 lb (68 kg) in nine months.

The plan

You don't have to eat only breakfast foods for dinner, although you can if you like. The idea is to switch the typical portions of dinner and breakfast, so you eat your largest meal of the day in the morning, have a smaller lunch and eat a light meal such as soup, salad or cereal in the evening. You should also have a morning and afternoon snack, and not eat anything after 6 p.m. Reverse dieters also drink lots of hot water with lemon slices.

There's no calorie counting as such, but the plan is generally high protein and low carbohydrate, and you must eat only whole unprocessed foods.

Exercise

Exercise and activity are encouraged but are not central to this weight-loss programme.

How it works

The science behind this method of weight loss is simple: calories consumed in the evening don't necessarily equal those consumed in the morning. The reason for this is that any food eaten in the morning, after a night's sleep, tends to be used for heat and immediate energy needs throughout the day, so it isn't as likely to be stored as fat. Food eaten in the evening, meanwhile, can accumulate as fat, it is claimed, because we don't burn it off as efficiently while we are sleeping. So on the Reverse Diet, you are advised to eat a small meal in the evening that is just enough to satisfy you.

There is certainly plenty of evidence to back up the importance of breakfast. Many studies have shown that breakfast eaters are slimmer than those who skip it, and a study by Addenbrooke's Hospital in Cambridge found that people who ate the biggest breakfast put on the least weight – even though they consumed the most food in an average day.

Who is it best for?

Lifestyle: You have leisurely mornings, perhaps you work from home or do shift work – either way, you have time to spare in the morning, so can sit down and enjoy the most important

DAILY MENU EXAMPLE	
Breakfast	Grilled chicken breast with boiled potatoes and green beans. Glass of hot water with lemon and a piece of fruit
Snack	Pot of cottage cheese and a piece of fruit
Lunch	Omelette made with two eggs, served with baked beans. Fruit salad topped with fresh low-fat cream. Hot water with lemon
Snack	Boiled egg and half a slice of wholemeal toast with unsalted butter or margarine
Dinner	Porridge with a handful of berries or sultanas or a small bowl of soup

meal of your day. You may also be single and less likely to prepare or sit down for the evening family meal.

Personality: You're a morning person who likes to be up and about at the crack of dawn. However, you are also a homebody who likes to spend the evenings relaxing at home, rather than out socializing.

Body shape: You tend to put on weight all over and feel generally heavier than you'd like to be.

PROS	CONS
• Unlike some restrictive diets, this will actually expand your food choices at most meals.	• For people already stressed in the morning, the Reverse Diet may be tough to stick to, particularly if you have kids to get out the door.
• This isn't a calorie-restricted diet. You won't feel hungry all the time.	• You probably won't want to make this a permanent lifestyle change – as only ever eating a starter in restaurants for dinner could become soul-destroying. Also, you would have to eat out before 6 p.m.
• The diet encourages a shift in thinking and food behaviour, which can help you combat long-standing, unhealthy eating habits.	
• No food groups are banned – instead it encourages well-rounded, nutritious meals that include foods from across the food groups.	• Some people are not morning eaters, plain and simple, and will find it impossible to eat a large breakfast.
• The evening meal in the Reverse Diet may be smaller than you're used to, but the idea is that if you start eating larger breakfasts and good-sized lunches, you won't feel as hungry in the evening.	• This diet doesn't pay close attention to calorie intake, opting instead to suggest "reasonable portions", which means you may be tempted to overeat.

Any health concerns?

There's no real scientific evidence to support the idea that calories consumed in the evening are less likely to be burnt off and will therefore be stored as fat. However, this diet is not restrictive and it doesn't ban any food groups, so it shouldn't lead to any health concerns, provided that you make sure your three meals contain a healthy mix of protein, carbs, fruit and vegetables.

The biggest obstacle to long-term weight loss is likely to be lifestyle, as society is unlikely to place breakfast above dinner in the near future – so, unless you can find a version that fits in with your evening routine, you may ultimately regain any weight loss. Still, the good news is there are no downsides to bigger breakfasts, as long as you are eating healthy foods.

Want to know more?

Read: *The Reverse Diet: Lose 20, 50, 100 Pounds or More by Eating Dinner for Breakfast and Breakfast for Dinner* by Tricia Cunningham and Heidi Skolnik (John Wiley & Sons, 2008).

The Scarsdale Diet

Two weeks of little but protein to ensure rapid weight loss.

The weight-loss promise:
"Lose up to 20 lb (9 kg) in 14 days."

Dr Tarnower

The Scarsdale Diet was one of the first high-protein, rapid weight-loss diets to become a craze. The plan itself was published in 1979 in the book *The Complete Scarsdale Medical Diet* by Dr Herman Tarnower, of Scarsdale, New York, who specialized in treating obesity. Its popularity benefited from a storm of publicity in 1980, when Dr Tarnower was murdered by his long-time lover, the headmistress of a well-known girls' boarding school.

The plan

Dr Tarnower wanted to create a diet that really helped his obese patients to lose weight and, most importantly, keep it off long-term. He proposed a strict low-calorie (850–1,000 calories a day) low-fat, low-carb plan, to be followed for 14 days. A less restrictive plan for 1–2 weeks then follows, known as the Keep Trim programme, before going back on the diet plan for another 14 days, if required.

The Scarsdale programme involves heavy consumption of protein. In fact, much of the diet consists of lean meats, plus salads, fruit and protein-rich bread. Breakfast is half a grapefruit and 1 slice of bread. Lunch may be fruit alone, or meat, fish or cheese with salad or vegetables. Dinner is meat or fish with vegetables. Snacks are limited to raw carrots and celery. Alcohol is forbidden, but you may drink tea, coffee, diet soft drinks and water. No potatoes, peas, beans (other than green beans) or lentils are allowed, and no pasta, rice or other grains – except for bread when specified.

Exercise

Dieters are recommended to walk 2 miles (3 km) per day.

How it works

It's a strictly calorie-controlled diet and one of the earliest high-protein plans on record. Dr Tarnower wanted to devise a plan that used the metabolic state of ketosis to trigger weight loss. Normally the body burns carbohydrates for fuel. Restricting these sends the body into ketosis, whereby it burns its own fat for fuel. A person in ketosis gets energy from ketones, little carbon fragments that are the fuel created by the breakdown of fat stores. Instead of relying on the carbohydrate-rich foods normally eaten for energy, the body's fat stores

DAILY MENU EXAMPLE	
Breakfast	½ grapefruit, 1 slice of wholemeal toast (no spreads or butter), coffee (no sugar or milk)
Lunch	Canned tuna, salad with oil-free dressing, coffee
Dinner	Roast lamb (with all visible fat removed), salad with lemon and vinegar dressing, coffee

PROS	CONS
• The menu plan is very specific, making it easy for the user to follow.	• There is a heavy emphasis on lean meats with most of the calories coming from animal-protein foods. It would be a difficult diet for vegetarians to follow.
• Rapid weight loss is appealing if you want to shape up for a holiday, party or other special event.	
• There's no portion control, so in theory you can eat as much as you want of one thing, as long as you stick to the plan.	• The cyclical style of the Scarsdale Diet plan is also difficult for many people, as there's a risk you will simply stop the diet at the end of the 14 days and regain all the weight you've lost.
• It's fairly easy to eat out, as you can just choose meat or fish and veg.	• In a state of ketosis, people often suffer from symptoms that include headaches, bad breath and constipation.

become the main energy source. When the body is in ketosis, you tend to feel less hungry and so are less likely to overeat.

The plan also includes eating half a grapefruit every day at breakfast for the supposed "fat burning enzyme" it contains. Tarnower said that this optimizes results because it prevents the metabolism from adjusting to the lower calorie intake.

Who is it best for?

Lifestyle: You have plenty of time to dedicate to planning, shopping and cooking meals, and you enjoy eating out and lots of meat. You may also have a holiday or other event coming up for which you'd like to look your best.

Personality: You love rules and relish the idea of a strict diet to take the guesswork out of trying to lose weight. You're also impatient and want fast results.

Body shape: Any, but this kind of plan is best for those with at least 2 stone (28 lb/13 kg) to lose.

Any health concerns?

Many dieters complain of fatigue and extreme hunger. The calorie level of 850–1,000 calories is too low for even a moderately active individual, and the plan shouldn't be undertaken without medical supervision. Most people would struggle to do the recommended amount of physical exercise, given the very low calorie intake. Following the Scarsdale Diet once for 14 days shouldn't put your health at risk unless you have an underlying health condition. However, it's dangerous to keep repeating the diet cycle, as it could lead to nutritional deficiencies in the long term. High-protein diets are not recommended for those with kidney problems, and have been linked to higher rates of kidney stones and osteoporosis.

Critics argue that you will only lose water weight and that you put it straight back on again as soon as you stop dieting. Some experts fear it promotes yo-yo dieting, generally considered bad for your health, and it may permanently affect your metabolism, making it harder to lose weight than before.

Want to know more?

Visit: www.scarsdale-diet-plan.com

The Six-Meals-a-Day Diet

Eating little and often, instead of the normal three meals a day, is the key to losing weight.

The weight-loss promise:
Lose up to 10 lb (4.5 kg) in the first 14 days – with no calorie counting, no starvation and no deprivation.

The origins of this diet philosophy are unclear, but some people believe it emerged out of the bodybuilding culture of the 1950s, when muscle men would eat little and often to keep their energy levels up.

It became well known as a weight-loss plan in the noughties, when a string of glamorous celebrities started claiming they kept their bodies red-carpet ready by eating six small meals a day. Actresses Jessica Biel, Eva Longoria and Charlize Theron are reportedly all fans.

After losing 40 lb (18 kg) by eating six mini meals a day, American fitness expert Jorge Cruise developed an eating plan based on the idea. He then wrote *The New York Times* bestselling diet book *The 3-Hour Diet*, which focuses on eating small meals, every three hours.

The plan

This diet sets itself up as the antithesis to low-carb weight-loss plans and encourages dieters to enjoy carbs and sweet treats every day. The focus of this plan is on when you eat, rather than what you eat.

You should eat breakfast within one hour of rising, eat every three hours thereafter and stop eating three hours before bedtime. Breakfast is at 7 a.m.; three hours later at 10 a.m. there's a 100-calorie snack. Three hours after your snack comes lunch, then three hours later another 100-calorie snack, followed in three hours by dinner. During, or soon after, dinner you enjoy a small 50-calorie treat. Your timing here should have you eating this last item three hours before bed. There's no eating after that.

Portion control is also important. According to Cruise, you should visualize what you're eating. Imagine a 9-in (23-cm) plate, on which you "see" four items:

• A Rubik's cube, representing your carbohydrate portion at breakfast, lunch and dinner.
• A deck of playing cards, symbolizing your protein serving at each meal; this is approximately 3oz (85 g). Cruise says it can be anything you like – from chicken to cheese, eggs and fish.
• A water-bottle cap represents the amount of fat on your plate – a little more than one teaspoon. This can be salad dressing, butter, olive oil – any fat you like.
• Visually stack three DVD cases; this represents how much fruit or vegetables to eat at each meal.

Cruise believes there are no bad foods, just bad portions. Using this "visual timing" method, he says you'll find that all meals are balanced at about 400 calories each. Cruise also advises drinking lots of water and taking a multivitamin every day.

Exercise

There is no exercise plan.

How it works

According to Cruise, eating every three hours will help you control your appetite, increase energy, preserve muscle, decrease belly size and burn fat through diet alone – hence the reason his book contains no exercise plan.

Cruise believes that eating frequent small meals teaches your body to constantly reset its metabolism, the theory being that since your body actually uses some calories to digest food, and digestion is a metabolic process, eating a meal theoretically "raises" your metabolism. So by eating frequently, you constantly keep your metabolism elevated.

DAILY MENU EXAMPLE	
Breakfast	1 hard-boiled egg, 1 slice wholegrain bread, salsa and a handful of watermelon cubes
Snack	12 cashews
Lunch	1 cheeseburger and side salad
Snack	24 cherries
Dinner	Beef and broccoli stir-fry with an apple, followed by 7 jellybeans
Desser	7 jellybeans

If you allow more than three hours to pass between meals, the theory holds, your body thinks that it's in "famine" mode and does everything it can to store the next available calories as fat, to ensure survival rather than burning them off. Eating every three hours also lessens belly fat, says Cruise, as regular

PROS	CONS
• Most calorie-restricted diets can leave you feeling hungry, but by eating six times a day, hunger is kept at bay.	• If you have trouble controlling the amount you eat at each meal, this diet may not be right for you, as the more times a day you sit down to eat a meal or snack, the more opportunities you have to overeat.
• You won't have to give up any of your favourite treats – there are no "bad" foods	
• Eating out is easy – even burgers are allowed!	• Eating more frequently could actually mean less nutrition and more calories if you don't carefully plan out your snacks and meals.
	• Making sure that healthy foods are to hand every three hours is very time-consuming.
	• Eating six mini meals a day can be a challenge when you're away from home, and some workplaces may not be conducive to this eating plan.

meals reduce levels of the stress hormone cortisol, which research shows can make your body store excess fat. Consistent eating is also said to keep blood-sugar levels stable, helping to suppress your appetite.

Cruise also stresses the importance of not placing restrictions on food options. He believes this is critical to successful weight loss because you will never need to cheat and thus sabotage your diet success.

Who is it best for?

Lifestyle: You're super-busy but super-scheduled during the working day, with a diary full of pre-planned appointments and meetings, which often means you're eating on the run. Preparing healthy mini meals in advance will help you fit a healthy diet into your hectic daily activities.

Personality: A reward seeker. You've always rewarded yourself with treats when things go well and comforted yourself when things go awry. This diet plan won't ban your goodies – it will just teach you to get them in proportion. You may also be a planner and something of a control freak – able to control both yourself and your schedule.

Body shape: Fairly slim but with a tummy and thighs, caused by serial snacking, that you'd like to trim. This plan should shift your focus from high-calorie snacks to balanced mini meals.

Any health concerns?

There are no real health concerns attached to this diet, as it doesn't involve cutting out any food groups. However, there is a real concern that planning to eat six times a day could actually lead some people to eat more calories than they were previously. In addition, as there are no "bad" foods, dieters could make unhealthy choices at mealtimes and fill up on sugary foods rather than nutrient-rich ones. Cruise simply assumes that people on his plan will show self-control and make good choices.

The underlying science is also shaky. A review in the *American Journal of Clinical Nutrition* concluded there was no real weight-loss advantage to eating six meals a day, while another study, in the *British Journal of Nutrition*, found no weight-loss difference between dieters who ate their calories in three meals a day or those who ate six meals.

Want to know more?

Read: *The 3-Hour Diet Cookbook* by Jorge Cruise (Collins, 2008).

The South Beach Diet

Swap "bad" carbs and fat for "good" carbs and fat to lose weight in a fortnight and improve your heart health for life.

The weight-loss promise:
Lose 8–13 lb (3.5–6 kg) in the next two weeks and lower your cholesterol, along with your risk of heart disease, diabetes and certain cancers.

The South Beach Diet was designed by cardiologist Arthur Agatston and dietician Marie Almon as an alternative to the popular low-fat approaches to weight loss and health.

While Agatston accepted the prevailing belief that a low-fat diet would reduce cholesterol and prevent heart disease, he found that patients had a hard time sticking to it. He was aware of the Atkins Diet but feared that it would lead to too few carbohydrates, too much saturated fat and too little fibre, so he set to work designing a new diet plan for his patients. While his main aim was to improve heart health, he discovered that, as a side effect, they also lost significant amounts of weight. In 2003, he outlined his diet plan in the best-selling book *The South Beach Diet* – named after the area in Miami where he lived.

When President Bill Clinton admitted to following the diet plan, it quickly gained widespread popularity and Agatston has since gone on to write many other South Beach Diet books.

The plan

There's no counting calories or rules about portion size – you simply eat three meals a day, and always until you're full. This diet is lower in carbohydrates and higher in protein and healthy fats than a typical healthy-eating plan, but it is not a strict low-carb diet. Instead of avoiding all carbs and fat, you simply have to differentiate between "good carbs" and "bad carbs", and "good fats" and "bad fats", and only eat the good variety of each.

Bad carbs are heavily refined sugars and grains, and high-GI (glycaemic index) foods that make up a large part of the typical Western diet. Good carbs are relatively unprocessed foods such as vegetables, beans and whole grains, which have a low GI. Bad fats are trans fats and saturated fats, while good fats are unsaturated fats and omega-3 fatty acids. Specifically, the diet excludes fatty red meat and poultry, replacing it with lean meats, nuts and oily fish. The diet is divided into three phases, each progressively becoming more liberal.

Phase 1: This lasts for two weeks and involves cutting out almost all carbohydrates from your diet, including pasta, rice, bread, baked goods and fruit. You can't drink fruit juice or any alcohol. A few low-GI, high-fibre vegetables such as broccoli and cabbage are allowed, but the focus is on eating lean protein, low-fat dairy, and foods with healthy unsaturated fats, including avocados, nuts and seeds.

Phase 2: For a following two weeks, you reintroduce low-GI carbs, including most fruits and vegetables, plus whole-grain breads, pasta and brown rice. Plus you can pick two items from the list of banned foods and reintroduce them as treats – for example, pasta or chocolate.

Phase 3: The maintenance phase, which lasts for life. There's no specific list of permitted and prohibited foods. Dieters are expected to take what they have learned and apply it to their life, including occasional indulgences.

Exercise

Dr Agatston recommends 20 minutes a day, alternating between interval training and normal exercise on a daily basis.

How it works

According to Agatston, food cravings are triggered not by carbohydrates in general but by carbohydrate-rich foods that the body digests quickly, creating a spike in blood sugar (high-GI foods). Such foods include heavily refined sugars and

DAILY MENU EXAMPLE	

Phase 1

Breakfast	Smoked salmon with scrambled eggs, vegetable juice
Mid-morning snack	Fat-free milk
Lunch	Summer vegetable salad with grilled scallop
Mid-afternoon snack	Nuts
Dinner	Pork and pepper salad with balsamic vinaigrette

PROS	CONS
• This diet is relatively easy to follow as you won't have to weigh out portion sizes or count calories.	• The extreme carbohydrate restriction in the first two weeks requires serious willpower and may leave you feeling weak and wobbly.
• After the first two weeks, the rest of the diet isn't very restrictive.	• In Phase 1 it is difficult to get your 5-a-day, which may leave you missing out on some vitamins and minerals.
• You should not go hungry on the South Beach Diet, as it promotes eating until you're full.	• The lack of guidance on portion sizes could lead you to overeat.
• It should banish cravings for sugary foods.	• To implement the diet changes permanently, you are left to your own devices, which could lead to the return of bad habits.

grains. Agatston believes that this is why people have a hard time sticking to low-fat diets that are still high in carbohydrates.

Agatston bans these foods for the first two weeks of his diet, which he says corrects the way your body reacts to them and puts an end to cravings for highly sugary foods. The weight loss doesn't happen because you're trying to eat less, but because you'll be eating fewer of the foods that created those former urges to eat more.

The South Beach Diet asserts that regular exercise will boost your metabolism and help prevent weight-loss plateaus. He recommends interval training – alternating short-burst, high-intensity exercise with rest periods. Just as a car uses more petrol when you brake and accelerate, interval training burns more calories than walking at a steady pace, Agatson says, "The higher the intensity of the exercise, the longer the afterburn; that is, you will continue to burn more fat and calories after you've completed your exercise session."

Who is it best for?

Lifestyle: Chaotic – you're looking for a long-term eating plan that will bring stability to your life rather than a quick-fix diet. You may also have set aside a few weeks to really kick-start the new you with a target date and weight in mind.

Personality: Hyperactive – you need a diet that's going to balance your blood sugar and have a calming effect.

Body shape: Thyroid type – naturally slim but puts on weight all over on the wrong diet. You often crave sugary foods, which this diet can help control.

Any health concerns?

A study in 2006 in the *Journal of General Internal Medicine* suggested that some of the health claims made by the South Beach Diet book were unsubstantiated. However, the diet itself is pretty healthy, being rich in vegetables, fruit, whole grains and lean protein. Most importantly, it doesn't leave out any major food groups. But experts note that, during Phase 1, much of the lost weight is water weight.

Health guidelines recommend losing no more than 2 lb (900 g) a week, so the fact that this diet promotes such a large weight loss – up to 13 lb (6 kg) – in the first two weeks could be deemed unhealthy and is probably just the result of a severe calorie restriction caused by cutting out all carbs. But once you get past the initial two weeks, provided that you implement the general guidelines in the long term, this is a nutritious, balanced diet.

Want to know more?

Read: *The South Beach Diet Supercharged* by Dr Arthur Agatston (Rodale, 2010).

The Sugar Addicts Diet

A plan for those with a sweet tooth, designed to break an addiction to sugary treats and control food cravings.

The weight-loss promise:
"A cutting edge programme that cures your type of sugar addiction and puts you back on the road to weight control and good health."

Dr Jacob Teitelbaum

Diet fads that banish fat or ditch carbs have been around for a long time, but in the last 10 years there have been many diets that choose to ban sugar. These plans all take the view that sugary foods can become uniquely addictive in a way that's closer to substances such as tobacco, alcohol and drugs than to other foodstuffs. And because sugary foods are so high in calories, this leads us to put on excess weight.

The official line has always been that, while sugar is high in calories, it's not addictive, but an increasing amount of research suggests the opposite may be true. One such study in 2002 at Princeton University in the US looked at the effects sugar had on chemicals in the brain. During the research, rats were fed a 25 per cent sugar solution – an amount equivalent to the sugar concentration of soft drinks – along with their normal food. After one month, the rats became "dependent" on the sugar solution, ate less food and increased their intake of the sugary drink by a startling 200 per cent.

Some experts now believe excess sugar could be a leading culprit in the rise in obesity and believe its use should be restricted. In 2003, a report commissioned by the World Health Organization and the Food and Agriculture Organization recommended that sugar should not account for more than 10 per cent of a person's diet. The idea behind most "sugar addict" diet plans, therefore, is to break this supposed sugar addiction so that you follow a healthier diet.

The plan

You'll have to give up all sugary foods and refined carbs, such as white bread, white rice and chips (fries), and replace them with high-fibre carbs. But it's not just obvious sweet foods like chocolate, cakes and fizzy drinks that need to be avoided – foods such as dips, cooking sauces, ketchup and yogurts contain hidden sugars and so are off limits, too. In addition, you're encouraged to eat plenty of "good" fats found in fish, nuts and seeds, to help burn the calories from carbs more quickly, along with some low-glycaemic carbohydrates in every meal. Many plans also encourage you to eat vegetables at every meal and, ideally, to stick to organic foods. Sugar-addiction theory aside, this way of eating has been described as a cross between the Mediterranean and Paleo Diets.

Exercise

Although there isn't a specific exercise plan with this diet, being generally more active is recommended. It's noted that when people work out, they often want to eat more healthily.

How it works

Although we need a certain amount of sugar in our diets to fuel our body and brain, large amounts have been linked with raised levels of the hormone insulin, which increases the risk of diabetes. The body also turns surplus sugar into fat, which is stored around the major vital organs, placing us at risk of liver and heart disease.

Sweets, sugary desserts and fizzy drinks are obvious culprits, but the anti-sugar brigade also sees carbohydrates, such as bread and pasta, as the enemy because the body breaks them down into simple sugars. When eaten alone, certain carbs can trigger the same surge-and-crash cycle of blood sugar that accompanies more obviously sugary foods.

Whether you call it an addiction, an eating disorder or simply a bad habit, there does appear to be evidence of unhealthy behaviour linked to sugary foods. People tend to

DAILY MENU EXAMPLE

Based on a person with a fairly average 33 points daily allowance

Breakfast	Scrambled eggs with red peppers, 1 slice whole-grain bread and a handful of strawberries
Snack	Handful of almonds
Lunch	Chicken and avocado salad
Snack	Houmous with carrot and celery sticks
Dinner	Salmon with mustard coating, with tomato rice salad and steamed asparagus

lose control and consume more sugar than they planned. They may also experience withdrawal symptoms if they skip their regular sugar "fix", the symptoms of which can include anxiety, shakiness or the jitters.

The various sugar-addict diets all claim that by breaking your addiction to sugar you'll prevent the swings in blood sugar that one minute leave you feeling euphoric and the next minute leave you craving another fix. This, in turn, will help you to lose weight because you'll no longer have the desire to snack constantly on sugary foods. In reality, the theory for this plan is similar to diets based on the glycaemic index (GI), which also regulate blood-sugar levels.

Who is it best for?

Lifestyle: Busy mums or professionals who often grab sweet snacks on the run to keep them going because they don't have time to stop and eat properly.

Personality: You have an addictive personality and find it hard to turn down that extra biscuit (cookie) or piece of chocolate, especially in moments of stress.

Body shape: You have a big tummy – the theory holds that sugar addiction can result in a tendency to store fat here.

Any health concerns?

Some sugar "detox diets" urge you to eliminate everything sweet – including fruit, dairy and all refined grains – to purge your system of sugar. But most experts agree that dietary changes this extreme tend to be too drastic to be sustained for any length of time. And research also shows that if you attempt

PROS	CONS
• It's not too extreme and is pretty healthy, encouraging the intake of fresh, unprocessed, organic foods.	• Some experts say that managing blood-sugar levels doesn't actually affect weight loss directly, so you may not see significant results unless you also cut your calorie intake.
• It may help wean you off sugary foods.	
• Because it focuses on regulating insulin production, it may help keep your blood sugar stable, reducing the associated food cravings and energy spikes and dips.	• You'll probably have to give up or strictly limit some of your favourite foods.
	• Quitting sugar cold turkey can produce unpleasant withdrawal symptoms such as headaches, fatigue and irritability.

to stay on a diet that is not sustainable, ultimately you risk going back to your old habits and putting any weight that you've lost straight back on – the classic yo-yo.

Nevertheless, when you strip away the fashionable language, the majority of sugar-addict diets are basically healthy-eating plans, with a good balance of lean protein, healthy fats, whole grains and fruit and veg. Provided you stick to it, you will probably experience weight loss.

Want to know more?

Read: *Beat Sugar Addiction Now!* by Dr Jacob Teitelbaum (Fair Winds Press, 2010).

WeightWatchers

Stick to your fixed daily points quota and – with a little help from your friends – you can eat the foods you like and still lose weight.

The weight-loss promise:
A steady weight loss of 2lb (900 g) a week.

The concept of WeightWatchers began in the early sixties when overweight housewife Jean Nidetch invited friends to her New York home to discuss how they could lose some weight. Together, they decided to follow a diet recommended by Jean's dietician, and began meeting regularly to chart their progress and swap tips. As the group expanded, Jean joined forces with businessman Al Lippert. WeightWatchers was born.

More than 40 years on, WeightWatchers International says it has helped millions of people all over the world to lose weight. There are around 7,000 meetings in the UK each week alone.

The WeightWatchers plan had been based on a food score points system, but in 2010 WeightWatchers controversially updated the points system with a new programme called ProPoints. Despite some backlash from devotees, science officer for WeightWatchers, Karen Miller-Kovach, describes ProPoints as simply a new approach to the same old safe, effective weight-loss plan: "With the old points system, you could use your points any way you like, but we now know if you use your points wisely by eating foods rich in protein and fibre, these foods fill you up, keep hunger at bay, and help you lose weight in a healthier and more nutritious way," she explained.

The plan

Based on your age, weight and other characteristics, you're assigned a daily ProPoints allowance, along with a weekly allowance. You then get to choose from a wide variety of healthy foods that you can split between three meals and snacks to make up your points allowance.

You're also encouraged to "maximize" your ProPoints allowance by choosing more "Power Foods", which include whole grains, lean meats, low-fat dairy and unlimited quantities of fresh fruit and non-starchy vegetables. Power Foods are the healthiest, most filling foods.

Decadent foods can still be worked into the points budget, but the new programme limits the amount of these extras. Dieters can check ProPoints values with a pocket guide that lists hundreds of the most popular foods, or online.

Exercise

Exercise is encouraged, and WeightWatchers assign a ProPoints value to a number of activities, such as swimming, dancing and even cleaning. Doing these activities counts as extra food points, which means you can enjoy an occasional food splurge. If you do an activity three or four times a week, for example, you can "spend" your extra points on a dinner out or a glass of wine.

How it works

You can eat whatever you want – provided you stick to your daily ProPoints target, a bespoke number based on your gender, weight, height and age. You can either do this alone or in a group by joining a weekly class.

The theory is that there's more to dieting than counting calories – if you make healthy choices that also fill you up, you'll eat less and feel better. The new WeightWatchers' ProPoints programme assigns every food a points value, based on its protein, carbohydrate, fat, fibre and calorie content, and how hard your body has to work to burn it off. Choices that fill you up the longest "cost" the least, and nutritionally dense foods cost less than empty calories. This means unhealthy choices such as burgers always have the highest point values and so should be eaten in small amounts or less often, while fresh fruits and vegetables carry zero points, so you can eat as many as you like, as often as you like.

By sticking to your points limit you will take in fewer calories and so lose weight. WeightWatchers hold weekly classes around the country, for which you pay a small fee to attend, in order to feel the support of a group of like-minded dieters. Weekly weigh-ins are an important part of these sessions – successful weight loss can be congratulated, so boosting your motivation to stick with the diet.

Who is it best for?

Lifestyle: You love a sense of order and rules and are pretty busy, so a system that requires little independent thought is perfect.

Personality: You're sociable and like sharing, so the idea of attending meetings, dieting with others and taking part in weekly weigh-ins is very motivating.

Body shape: You carry excess weight all over and have at least 2 stone (28 lb/13 kg) you want to shift.

Based on a person with a fairly average 33 points daily allowance

Breakfast	Fat-free Greek yogurt pot with low-sugar muesli and fresh strawberries
Snack	Latte with skimmed milk
Lunch	Grilled chicken with salad of cherry tomatoes, carrots, lettuce and low-fat dressing
Snack	Microwave popcorn
Dinner	Stir-fry prawns (shrimp) with garlic, brown rice and steamed mixed vegetable

Any health concerns?

Some critics think the WeightWatchers points system makes losing weight more complicated than it really is. After all, if you eat fewer calories than you burn off, you will lose weight – it's that simple. These critics argue that it's vital that people actually learn how many calories are in foods and how this contributes to their energy needs, rather than just attributing points to foods because, in the long term, this deeper knowledge will be what helps people keep the weight off.

PROS	CONS
• No foods are banned – in fact, treating yourself is encouraged, so you won't feel deprived of your favourite foods.	• Some long-term members, who were familiar with the old pre-2010 points system, have complained of slow weight loss under the revised plan.
• You won't go hungry – daily points are always high enough to allow for three meals a day, plus at least two snacks.	• Some dieticians argue that fruit shouldn't be "free" food for someone who is trying to lose weight, as it can be high in calories.
• Some studies suggest WeightWatchers is effective.	• It can take time to learn the points system, and the need to research the point score of every food you eat can be tiresome.

A criticism of the old system was that you could, in theory, use up all of your points eating only chocolate, if you so chose. The new ProPoints programme addresses this long-term problem by steering people to make healthier choices. For example, all veg are given zero points to encourage people to eat more. WeightWatchers recommends taking a daily multivitamin, an admission that people left to make their own food choices could miss out on certain important nutrients.

Want to know more?

Visit: www.weightwatchers.co.uk or www.weightwatchers.com

The Zone Diet

Get in the "zone" with an insulin-regulating low-carb plan and your health will benefit while the pounds drop off.

The weight-loss promise:
You could lose at least 5 lb (2.25 kg) in the first two weeks, followed by 1–1½ lb (0.5–0.7 kg) every week thereafter.

According to Dr Barry Sears, the creator of this popular Hollywood diet, the "Zone" is a place where we find ourselves "feeling alert, refreshed and full of energy". Sears, a former scientist, claims that as well as enjoying weight loss by following his Zone diet, you can also reduce your risk of heart disease, high blood pressure and diabetes.

Like other low-carb plans, his diet, created in 1995, dismisses the traditional thinking about good nutrition – i.e. that we should follow a diet low in fats and protein but high in carbohydrates – as "dead wrong". He goes on to claim that this type of diet has actually contributed to our risk of becoming obese and contracting serious diseases, and that by changing to a lower-carb, higher-protein plan you can shed pounds and live longer.

The plan

The Zone doesn't recommend that you eat fewer calories than you're currently consuming, just different ones. Sears is rigid about sticking to the 40:30:30 ratio of protein, fat and carbohydrates that he feels each of us needs, and he encourages dieters to base the specific amounts on their own individual size, age and daily activity. Although his plan follows complex measurements of what to eat and when, it can be roughly simplified as:

- Eat a small amount of lean protein, such as chicken or fish, at every meal (approximately the size of your palm or one small chicken breast) and also for every snack (one in the late afternoon, one in the late evening).
- Eat "favourable" carbohydrates with every meal. These include most fruit and vegetables, lentils, beans and whole grains. This should be double the size of your protein portion.
- If you chose "unfavourable" carbs with your meal – a group that includes brown rice, pasta, papaya, mango, banana, dry breakfast cereal, bread, bagel, tortilla, carrots, and all fruit juices – you can only eat around half the portion size.
- For dairy, you should stick to low-fat or no-fat cheeses and milk. You're also encouraged to enjoy olive oil, nuts and avocados for their healthy fats. Junk and processed foods are discouraged.

Exercise

The Zone doesn't recommend a specific workout, but it does encourage regular physical activity (3–4 times per week) and suggests eating a zone snack 30 minutes before working out, to maximize the diet's effects.

DAILY MENU EXAMPLE	
Breakfast	Egg white and asparagus omelette cooked in olive oil, with fresh strawberries
Lunch	Chicken breast and mixed salad greens with tomato and olive oil salad dressing. Sliced pear
Dinner	Salmon poached in orange juice with pumpkin and courgette (zucchini) sautéed in butter. Blueberries

How it works

The Zone diet works on the theory that excess insulin, a hormone that helps control our blood sugar levels, makes us fat and keeps us fat. By closely regulating our blood-sugar levels, keeping our levels of insulin in a tight "zone", the body burns fat more efficiently so that we lose weight.

To control blood-sugar levels, and consequently insulin levels, Sears believes that you need to get the perfect balance of carbohydrates, proteins and fats in every meal. Achieving this perfect balance means following a low-carbohydrate, high-protein diet that includes moderate amounts of fat.

The ratio Sears claims the body is genetically programmed to favour is 40:30:30, where the 40 represents protein. Sears also suggests that we think of food not as a source of calories but "as a control system for our hormones".

PROS	CONS
• It has fewer dietary restrictions than many other low-carb plans.	• It can be very complicated and time-consuming if you follow it properly. You"ll need to invest in a Zone Diet book and a decent set of measuring scales and spoons.
• It recommends eating more fruit and vegetables.	
• It also encourages you to cut out a lot of the "junk" or low-nutrient carbs in your diet such as crisps (potato chips), cakes, biscuits (cookies) and chocolate.	• It can be very expensive – especially if you decide to purchase the pre-packaged "Zone" food products on sale in the US.
	• If you're counting the suggested "food blocks" in the book to work out allowable meal ratios, eating out could become akin to a hardcore maths class.

Who is it best for?

Lifestyle: Singletons with stress-free lives and time to focus just on food – trying to get your head around the "zones" of carbohydrate, protein and fat after a busy day in the office or chasing after the kids is just not going to happen!

Personality: You have a scientific mindset and enjoy complex theories and plans. You're also very disciplined and able to stick to strict rules.

Body shape: The Zone is another good diet for big tummies, as it reduces high-sugar food and claims to control blood-sugar levels, thereby reducing tummy fat and lowering heart disease risk.

Any health concerns?

A lot of experts question the science behind Sears' theory, arguing there is no real proof that the hormone insulin plays such a large role in weight control. This doesn't mean that Sears' theories are necessarily wrong – it's just that there is currently no robust scientific evidence to prove that his thinking is correct. Some nutritionists are also concerned that the recommended protein levels could be too high, especially for people with underlying health problems such as kidney disease.

The Zone Diet also recommends eliminating some very nutritious foods that are a good source of energy and also packed with fibre and important vitamins and minerals. For example, brown rice and other whole-grain cereals are off limits yet they're packed with fibre, B vitamins and iron, while full-fat cheese is good source of calcium and zinc.

Compared to other low-carb, high-protein plans, however, the Zone is probably a more balanced and sustainable approach – but only if you can get to grips with the 40:30:30 eating regime.

Want to know more?

Read: *The Zone Diet* by Dr Barry Sears (Thorsons, 2011).

Directory

On the following pages you will find recommended health and weight guidelines and eating plans. The chart below is based on National Health guidelines for the UK, while the chart on the facing page is based on guidelines from the US Department of Health and Human Services.

UK

Your weight in kilograms

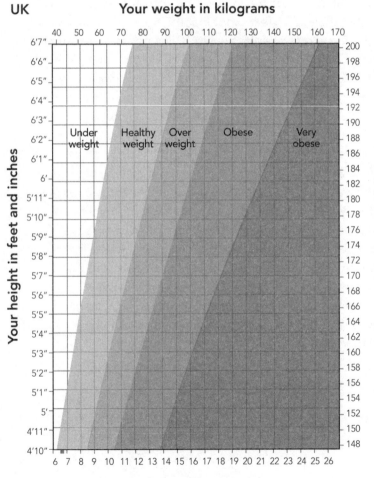

Your height in feet and inches

Your height in centimetres

Under weight   Healthy weight   Over weight   Obese   Very obese

Your weight in stones

BMI	19	20	21	22	23	24	25	26	27	28	29	30	31	32	33	34	35
Height							Weight in pounds										
4'10"	91	96	100	105	110	115	119	124	129	134	138	143	148	153	158	162	167
4'11"	94	99	104	109	114	119	124	128	133	138	143	148	153	158	163	168	173
5'	97	102	107	112	118	123	128	133	138	143	148	153	158	163	168	174	179
5'1"	100	106	111	116	122	127	132	137	143	148	153	158	164	169	174	180	185
5'2"	104	109	115	120	126	131	136	142	147	153	158	164	169	175	180	186	191
5'3"	107	113	118	124	130	135	141	146	152	158	163	169	175	180	186	191	197
5'4"	110	116	122	128	134	140	145	151	157	163	169	174	180	186	192	197	204
5'5"	114	120	126	132	138	144	150	156	162	168	174	180	186	192	198	204	210
5'6"	118	124	130	136	142	148	155	161	167	173	179	186	192	198	204	210	216
5'7"	121	127	134	140	146	153	159	166	172	178	185	191	198	204	211	217	223
5'8"	125	131	138	144	151	158	164	171	177	184	190	197	203	210	216	223	230
5'9"	128	135	142	149	155	162	169	176	182	189	196	203	209	216	223	230	236
5'10"	132	139	146	153	160	167	174	181	188	195	202	209	216	222	229	236	243
5'11"	136	143	150	157	165	172	179	186	193	200	208	215	222	229	236	243	250
6'	140	147	154	162	169	177	184	191	199	206	213	221	228	235	242	250	258
6'1"	144	151	159	166	174	182	189	197	204	212	219	227	235	242	250	257	265
6'2"	148	155	163	171	179	186	194	202	210	218	225	233	241	249	256	264	272
6'3"	152	160	168	76	184	192	200	208	216	224	232	240	248	256	264	272	279
	Healthy Weight						Overweight					Obese					

You may find the two portion-control diagrams below helpful in maintaining your correct weight for your height. Both highlight the different types of food we eat and the proportions we should eat them in to have a well-balanced and healthy diet. The MyPlate, below, is the nutritional guide published by the United States Department of Agriculture; the Eatwell plate, on the facing page, is recommended by the UK Department of Health.

US MyPlate

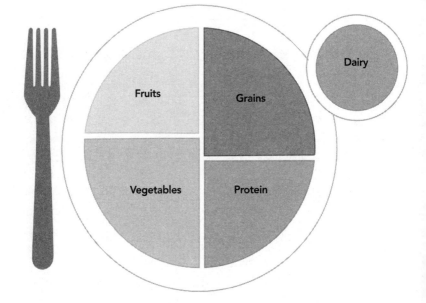

UK Eatwell Plate

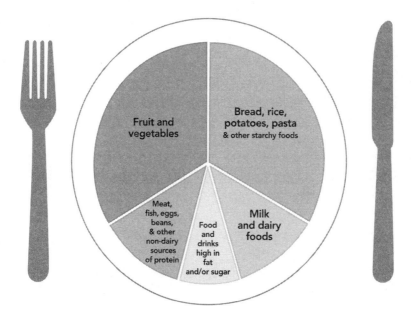